Basic Clinical
Pharmacokinetics

Basic Clinical Pharmacokinetics

Michael E. Winter, Pharm.D.
Associate Clinical Professor of Pharmacy
School of Pharmacy
University of California, San Francisco
and
Co-Director
Clinical Pharmacokinetics Laboratory
University of California Hospitals and Clinics
San Francisco

with
Brian S. Katcher, Pharm.D.
Lecturer in Pharmacy
School of Pharmacy
University of California, San Francisco

Mary Anne Koda-Kimble, Pharm.D.
Associate Clinical Professor of Pharmacy
Vice Chairwoman, Division of Clinical Pharmacy
School of Pharmacy
University of California, San Francisco

Applied Therapeutics, Inc.
San Francisco

Applied Therapeutics, Inc.
P.O. Box 31-747
San Francisco, CA 94131

Library of Congress catalog card number 80-69785
ISBN 0-915486-04-0

Published December 1980
First Printing

Contents

Expanded Contents

1. Basic Principles *(continued)*

1. Basic Principles *(continued)*

Part Two

2. Digoxin 71

3. Lidocaine 93

3. Lidocaine *(continued)*

6. Theophylline *(continued)*

xiii

Introduction

In recent years, the evaluation of drug concentrations in biological fluids has gained increased acceptance as a guide for monitoring drug therapy. Pharmacokinetics and biopharmaceutics are useful in predicting plasma drug concentrations as well as changes in plasma drug concentrations which occur over time. This book is divided into two parts. The first reviews basic pharmacokinetic principles and the second illustrates the clinical application of pharmacokinetics to specific drugs through the presentation and solution of sample problems which are commonly encountered in the practice setting.

Part One is divided into sections which describe major pharmacokinetic parameters and their clinical applications. Equations which express the relationships between the various parameters are presented and discussed.[1] The reader is strongly urged to read each section in the order that it appears in the text because many of the concepts discussed in the latter portion of Part One are based upon an understanding of those presented earlier.

Many individuals feel overwhelmed by the apparent complexity of some of the equations used to describe the pharmacokinetic behavior of drugs. Therefore, extensive explanations which emphasize major concepts accompany the more complex equations. Figures to help the reader visualize the concepts have also been included throughout the text. The principles discussed in Part One were selected to give the clinician a basis for interpreting plasma drug concentrations and manipulating the dosage regimens for the drugs discussed in Part Two of this text.

The drugs discussed in Part Two of this text were selected because their clinical assays are widely available and because an understanding of their pertinent pharmacokinetic and biopharmaceutic properties can substantially aid clinicians in dosing

---

1. Some mathematical assumptions were made to predict plasma levels and to adjust dosing regimens. This is common practice in the actual clinical setting. A more detailed and in-depth discussion of pharmacokinetic principles and their mathematical derivations can be found elsewhere (1,43,224).

them more rationally and safely. A method of calculating a loading and maintenance dose for each drug is discussed. In addition, pathophysiologic factors which influence the pharmacokinetics of these drugs and their significance are considered.

Although plasma levels are useful in evaluating therapy, they constitute only one monitoring parameter and should, therefore, not be used as the sole criterion on which treatment is based. Pharmacokinetic calculations should only be considered a guide to the determination of dosage regimens.

If a calculated dosage regimen seems unreasonable, re-evaluation is essential since mathematical error is always a possibility. Another problem inherent in these calculations is that the pharmacokinetic parameters utilized may be inappropriate for the patient under consideration. Many of the pharmacokinetic parameters available in the literature are based on small numbers of patients or on normal volunteers (38,41,52). Therefore, values obtained from these experimental data are, at best, estimates for any given patient. If the basic underlying pharmacokinetic assumptions are not applicable to a particular patient, even the most elegant calculation is invalid.

Review articles commonly list pharmacokinetic parameters for a number of drugs (2,25,41); however, the reader is encouraged to seek out the original literature to evaluate the methodology and data from which this information was derived.[2] Some factors which should be considered in scrutinizing these studies include the number and type of subjects, type and specificity of drug assay, degree of inter-subject variability, statistical analysis of the data, and whether the study was done prospectively or retrospectively. These problems emphasize the need to obtain accurate plasma-level measurements as well as the need to re-evaluate the appropriateness of pharmacokinetic parameters for each patient (12).

---

2. A recently published text reviews the pharmacokinetic literature for a large number of drugs: *Applied Pharmacokinetics: Principles of Therapeutic Drug Monitoring* edited by W.E. Evans, J.J. Schentag and W.J. Jusko, Applied Therapeutics, Inc., San Francisco, 1980.

PART ONE

1

Basic Principles

BIOAVAILABILITY (F)

Bioavailability is the percentage or fraction of the administered dose which reaches the systemic circulation of the patient. To calculate the amount of drug absorbed, the administered dose should be multiplied by a bioavailability factor, which is usually represented by the letter "F." For example, the bioavailability of digoxin is estimated to be 0.62 for orally administered tablets (31). This means that if 250 mcg (0.25 mg) of digoxin is given orally, the effective or absorbed dose (155 mcg) can be calculated by multiplying the administered dose by F:

$$(F)(Dose) = \text{Amt. of Drug Absorbed or} \atop \text{Amt. of Drug Reaching the Systemic Circulation} \qquad \text{(Eq. 1)}$$

(0.62)(250 mcg) = 155 mcg

It should be emphasized that this factor does not take into consideration the *rate* of drug absorption; it only estimates the *extent* of absorption. Although the rate of absorption can be important when a rapid onset of drug action is required, it is not usually important when a drug is administered chronically. Rate of absorption becomes important only if it is so slow that it limits the absolute bioavailability of the drug. This occasionally occurs with some sustained release preparations (3).

There are a number of factors which must be considered when estimating the bioavailability of a drug. Bioavailability can vary among different formulations and **dosage forms** of a drug. For example, digoxin elixir appears to have a bioavailability of approximately 77% (F = 0.77) as compared to the tablets which have a bioavailability of 62% (F = 0.62) (31). When drugs are given parenterally, the bioavailability is usually considered to be 100% (F = 1.0). By rearranging Eq.1, this principle can be used to calculate equivalent doses of a drug when a patient is switched from one dosage form to another.

$$\frac{\text{Dose of New}}{\text{Dosage Form}} = \frac{\substack{\text{Amt. of Drug Absorbed from} \\ \text{Current Dosage Form}}}{\text{F of New Dosage Form}} \qquad \text{(Eq. 2)}$$

For example, let us assume that a patient who has been receiving daily doses of 250 mcg (0.25 mg) of digoxin as the tablet is to be switched to an elixir. An equivalent dose of the elixir would be calculated as follows:

$$\text{Dose of Elixir} = \frac{155 \text{ mcg}}{0.77}$$

$$= 201 \text{ mcg}$$

The **chemical form** in which a drug is administered must also be considered. For example, when a salt or ester of a drug is administered, the bioavailability factor, or F, should be multiplied by the fraction of the total molecular weight which the active drug represents. If "S" represents the fraction of the administered dose which is the active drug, then the amount of drug absorbed from a salt or ester form can be calculated as follows:

$$(S)(F)(Dose) = \substack{\text{Amt. of Drug Absorbed or} \\ \text{Amt. Reaching the Systemic Circulation}} \qquad \text{(Eq. 3)}$$

The "S" factor should be included in all bioavailability equations as a constant reminder of its importance in assessing bioavailability of the active drug form. When a drug is administered in its parent form, the "S" for that drug is 1.0.

Aminophylline is an excellent example of this principle. (See Fig. 1.) Aminophylline is the ethylenediamine salt of the pharmacologically active moiety, theophylline. Eighty to eighty-five percent (by weight) of this salt is theophylline, so that "S" for aminophylline is 0.8. Uncoated aminophylline tablets are considered to be completely (100%) available; the F or bioavailability factor for this dosage form is, therefore, 1.0. It is clear from this example that it is critical to consider the salt form in determining the amount of theophylline absorbed from an aminophylline tablet. When Eq. 3 is applied to this situation, it can be demonstrated that 160 mg of theophylline is absorbed from a 200 mg aminophylline tablet.

$$(0.8)(1.0)(200 \text{ mg Aminophylline}) = 160 \text{ mg Theophylline}$$

Finally, since drugs are absorbed from the gastrointestinal tract into the portal circulation, some drugs may be extensively metabolized in the liver before they reach the systemic circulation. This **"first-pass effect"** may substantially decrease the amount of active drug reaching the systemic circulation and thus, its bioavailability. See Fig. 2.

Lidocaine is an example of a drug with a first-pass effect that is so great that oral administration is not practical (23). In the case of propranolol, a significant portion of the orally administered dose is metabolized through a first-pass effect; therefore, a much larger oral dose is required to achieve the same pharmacologic response as that obtained from a dose administered intravenously. However, the propranolol issue is further complicated by the fact that one of the metabolites, 4-hydroxypropranolol, is pharmacologically active (39).

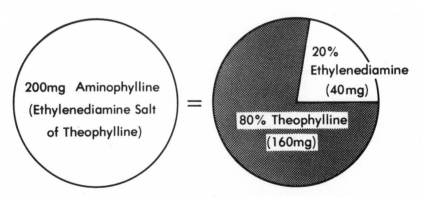

Fig. 1. The Effect of the Chemical Drug Form on Bioavailability. The example above emphasizes the need to consider the fraction of the chemical form administered which actually represents active drug when calculating the amount of drug administered. The bioavailability of the dosage form itself must also be considered when drugs are administered by the oral route.

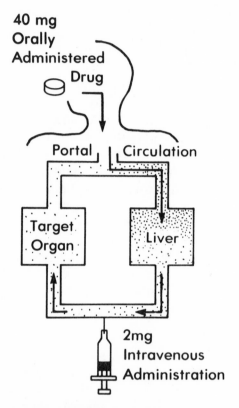

Fig. 2. First Pass Effect. When drugs with a high "first pass effect" are administered orally, a large amount of the absorbed drug is metabolized before it reaches the systemic circulation. If the drug is administered intravenously, the liver is by-passed, thereby increasing the fraction of the administered dose which reaches the circulation. Parenteral doses for drugs with a high first pass are much smaller than oral doses which produce equivalent pharmacologic effects.

ADMINISTRATION RATE (R$_A$)

The administration rate is the average rate at which the absorbed drug reaches the systemic circulation. This is usually calculated by dividing the amount of drug absorbed (see Eq. 3) by the time over which the drug was administered, or the dosing interval. The dosing interval is usually represented by the symbol for tau (τ).

$$\text{Administration Rate} \ (R_A) = \frac{(S)(F)(Dose)}{\tau} \qquad \text{(Eq. 4)}$$

When drugs are administered as a continuous infusion, tau can be expressed in any convenient time unit. For example, the theophylline administration rate resulting from aminophylline infused at a rate of 75 mg every hour is calculated from Eq. 4 as follows:

$$R_A = \frac{(0.8)(1.0)(75 \ mg)}{1 \ hour} = 60 \ mg/hour$$

$$R_A = \frac{(0.8)(1.0)(75 \ mg)}{60 \ minutes} = 1 \ mg/minute$$

When drugs are administered at fixed dosing intervals, the calculated administration rate is an average value. For example, the average administration rate of theophylline in mg/hr resulting from an oral dose of 300 mg aminophylline given every six hours would be calculated using Eq. 4 as follows:

$$R_A = \frac{(0.8)(1.0)(300 \ mg)}{6 \ hours} = 40 \ mg/hour$$

DESIRED PLASMA CONCENTRATION (Cp)

In the clinical setting, the drug concentration in plasma (Cp) which is reported by the laboratory represents drug that is bound to plasma protein plus drug that is unbound or free. It is the free or unbound form of the drug which is in equilibrium with the receptor site and is, therefore, the pharmacologically active moiety. Thus, the reported plasma drug concentration

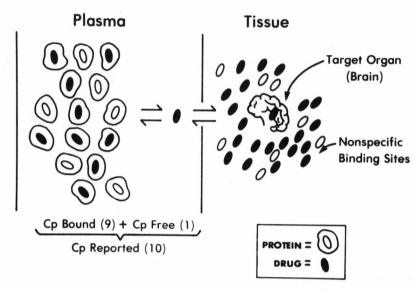

Fig. 3. Plasma Concentration of a Highly Protein-bound Drug: Normal Plasma Protein Concentration. Note that the plasma drug concentration reported by the laboratory represents a total of both "bound" and "free" drug. It is the "free" form which is in equilibrium with the target organs and is the pharmacologically active moiety. In this illustration alpha, or the fraction of free drug to total drug concentration is 0.1.

indirectly reflects the concentration of free or active drug. See Fig. 3.

Some disease states are associated with decreased plasma proteins or with decreased binding of drugs to plasma proteins (5). In these situations, drugs which are usually highly protein bound have a larger percent of free or unbound drug present in plasma. Therefore, a greater pharmacological effect can be expected for any given drug concentration in plasma (Cp). Clinicians must always consider altered protein binding and whether the **fraction of free drug concentration (alpha or "α")** is altered when interpreting or establishing desired plasma drug concentrations.

$$\alpha = \frac{\text{Free drug concentration}}{\text{Total drug concentration}} = \frac{\text{Cp free}}{\text{Cp bound} + \text{Cp free}} \qquad \text{(Eq. 5)}$$

In most cases, the fraction of drug which is free (α) does not vary with the drug concentration because the number of protein binding sites far exceeds the number of drug molecules available for binding and protein binding sites for drugs are seldom saturated. Two major factors control alpha: the plasma protein concentration (in many cases this is albumin) and the binding affinity of the drug for plasma protein.

Low plasma protein concentrations will decrease the concentration of bound drug (Cp bound) but generally not that of the free drug (Cp free). Therefore, alpha increases as plasma protein concentrations decrease. Free drug concentrations are not altered to a significant extent because the free drug which is released into plasma secondary to low plasma protein concentrations equilibrates with the tissue compartment (See Fig. 4 and compare with Fig. 3). Therefore, if the volume of distribution (Vd) is relatively large, only a minor increase in Cp free will result. Also see section on Volume of Distribution.

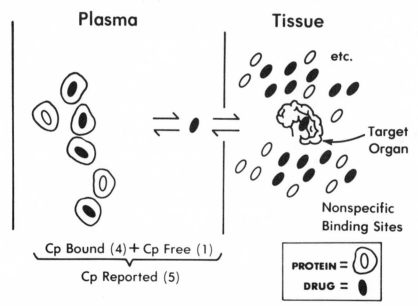

Plasma　　　　**Tissue**

etc.

Target Organ

Nonspecific Binding Sites

Cp Bound (4) + Cp Free (1)

Cp Reported (5)

PROTEIN = ⓪

DRUG = ●

Fig. 4. Effect of Decreased Plasma Protein Concentration on Plasma Drug Concentration. Compare this figure with Fig. 3. Note that the decreased protein concentration decreases the plasma drug concentration reported by the laboratory. In this situation, the concentration of free or active drug remains the same because free drug which is released into the plasma as a result of the lowered protein concentration is taken up by nonspecific binding sites. For this reason, the pharmacologic effect which can be expected from the reported Cp of 5 will be the same as that produced by the reported Cp of 10 in Fig. 3. In this illustration, alpha or the fraction of free drug to total drug concentration is increased to 0.2.

The relationship between the plasma drug concentration and the plasma protein concentration can be expressed as follows:

$$\frac{Cp'}{Cp \text{ adjusted}} = (1-\alpha) \left(\frac{P'}{P} \right) + \alpha \qquad \text{(Eq. 6)}$$

This equation can be used to estimate to what degree an altered plasma protein concentration will affect the desired therapeutic drug concentration. Cp' represents the plasma drug concentration and P' the plasma protein concentration in the patient. Cp adjusted, P and α are the plasma drug concentration, plasma protein concentration, and alpha that would be expected if the plasma protein concentration were normal. To calculate the Cp adjusted for any given drug, Eq. 6 can be rearranged to:

$$Cp \text{ adjusted} = \frac{Cp'}{(1-\alpha) \left(\dfrac{P'}{P} \right) + \alpha} \qquad \text{(Eq. 7)}$$

For example, a patient with a low serum albumin of 2.0 gm/dl (normal albumin 4.0 gm/dl) and an apparently low plasma phenytoin concentration of 5.5 mcg/ml still has a therapeutically acceptable plasma drug concentration when it is adjusted for the low serum albumin. When the normal α for phenytoin (0.1) is substituted into Eq. 7, an adjusted phenytoin plasma concentration of 10 mcg/ml can be calculated:

$$Cp \text{ adjusted} = \frac{Cp'}{(1-\alpha) \left(\dfrac{P'}{P} \right) + \alpha} \qquad \text{(Eq. 7)}$$

$$= \frac{5.5 \text{ mcg/ml}}{(1-0.1) \left(\dfrac{2 \text{ gm/dl}}{4 \text{ gm/dl}} \right) + 0.1}$$

$$= \frac{5.5 \text{ mcg/ml}}{(0.9)(0.5) + 0.1}$$

$$= \frac{5.5 \text{ mcg/ml}}{0.55} = 10 \text{ mcg/ml}$$

The Cp that would have been reported from the laboratory if the albumin had been "normal" would be approximately 10 mcg/ml. This calculation is based upon the assumption that phenytoin is primarily bound to albumin.

Many other drugs are not primarily bound to globulin rather than albumin. Adjustments for these drugs based upon serum albumin concentrations would therefore be inappropriate. Unfortunately, adjustments for changes in globulin binding are difficult because drugs usually bind to a specific globulin which is only a small fraction of total globulin concentration. In general, acidic drugs such as phenytoin and the barbiturates bind primarily to albumin, while basic drugs such as lidocaine and quinidine bind more extensively to the globulins (5,8,9,15,20).

When a patient's serum albumin concentration is elevated or only moderately low it is generally unnecessary to consider adjustment of the Cp by use of Eq. 7. The alpha value (fraction of free to total drug concentration) for selected drugs is provided in Table 1.

Table 1
DRUGS AND ALPHA VALUES FOR PLASMA PROTEIN BINDING

Drug	Alpha Value
Amitriptyline	0.04*
Chlordiazepoxide	0.05
Chlorpropamide	0.04
Chlorpromazine	0.04
Diazepam	0.01
Diazoxide	0.09
Digoxin	0.70
Digitoxin	0.10
Imipramine	0.04*
Lidocaine	0.30*
Methadone	0.13*
Nafcillin	0.10
Nortriptyline	0.06*
Phenylbutazone	0.01
Phenytoin	0.10
Propranolol	0.06*
Quinidine	0.20*
Salicylic Acid	0.16
Thiopental	0.13
Warfarin	0.03

*Basic drugs that are bound significantly to plasma proteins other than albumin.
Adapted from references 5, 8, and 9.

In contrast to low plasma protein concentrations, it is rarely necessary to consider *elevated* levels of plasma protein in the interpretation of plasma drug concentrations. However, quinidine is a notable exception. Increased concentrations of quinidine resulting from increased levels of quinidine binding proteins have been observed in patients who were recently stressed (e.g., surgery). When the concentration of binding protein is increased, the fraction of free to total drug concentration (α) decreases and free drug concentration remains the same due to re-equilibration with larger tissue stores. In this situation, one would anticipate that therapeutic levels of free or unbound drug would correlate with a reported drug concentration (bound plus free) which is higher than usual.

The **binding affinity** of plasma protein for a drug can also alter alpha, or the fraction of drug which is free. See Fig. 5 and compare with Fig. 3. For example, the plasma proteins in patients with uremia (severe renal failure) have less affinity for phenytoin than do proteins present in non-uremics. This is reflected by the fact that the alpha for phenytoin in uremic patients is estimated to be in the range of 0.2 to 0.3 in contrast to the normal value of 0.1 (20,40). The "effective" or free drug concentration can be obtained by simple rearrangement of Eq. 5:

$$\alpha = \frac{\text{Cp free}}{\text{Cp bound} + \text{Cp free}} \qquad \text{(Eq. 5)}$$

$$= \frac{\text{Cp free}}{\text{Cp total}}$$

Cp free = (α)(**Cp total**)   (Eq. 8)

It is evident from Eq. 8 that as a result of the increased alpha for phenytoin in uremic patients, lower phenytoin plasma concentrations (Cp total) will achieve free drug concentrations comparable to those attained in non-uremic patients. For example, a uremic patient with an alpha of 0.25 and a reported phenytoin concentration of 4 mcg/ml would have the same free drug concentration (same pharmacologic effect) as a patient with normal renal function and a reported phenytoin concentration of 10 mcg/ml:

Plasma   Tissue

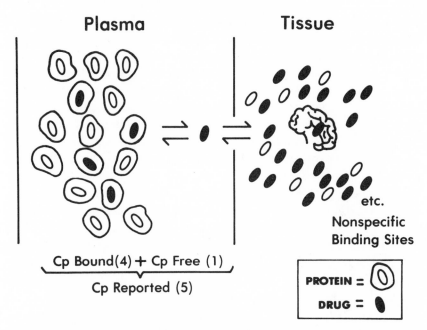

Cp Bound(4) + Cp Free (1)

Cp Reported (5)

etc.

Nonspecific Binding Sites

PROTEIN =

DRUG =

Fig. 5. The Effect of Decreased Binding Affinity on Plasma Drug Concentration. Compare this figure with Fig. 3. Note that even though the protein concentration is normal, the decreased binding affinity of the drug for protein has decreased the reported drug concentration. The concentration of free or active drug remains the same because free drug which is released into the plasma as a result of this decreased affinity is taken up by nonspecific binding sites in the tissue. Thus, the pharmacologic effect which can be expected from the reported Cp of 5 will be the same as that produced by the reported Cp of 10 in Fig. 3. In this illustration, alpha or the fraction of free drug to total drug concentration is increased to 0.2.

$$\text{Cp free} = (\alpha)(\text{Cp total}) \qquad \text{(Eq. 8)}$$

$$\text{Cp free in uremic patient} = (0.25)(4 \text{ mcg/ml})$$

$$= 1.0 \text{ mcg/ml}$$

$$\text{Cp free in patient with normal renal function} = (0.1)(10 \text{ mcg/ml})$$

$$= 1.0 \text{ mcg/ml}$$

In summary, any factor which alters protein binding becomes clinically important when a drug is highly protein bound (i.e., if alpha is less than 0.1 or 10% free). For these drugs, even small changes in the fraction bound can substantially increase the amount of free drug available to pharmacologically active sites. For example, if as the result of decreased amounts of protein, α is increased from 0.1 (10% free) to 0.2 (20% free), the concentration of free, active drug available for any given value for Cp (total, bound and free) would double. If, on the other hand, the alpha for a drug is greater than or equal to 0.5 (50% free), it is unlikely that changes in plasma protein binding will be of clinical consequence. As an illustration, if the alpha for a drug increases from 0.5 (50% free) to 0.6 (60% free) as a result of decreased protein concentrations, the concentration of free, active drug, assuming the same total concentration, would actually be increased by only 20%.

As a general rule, if alpha increases in any given situation, the clinician should reduce the desired Cp by the same proportion (5). That is, if alpha is increased two-fold, the desired Cp should be reduced to one-half the usual value.

VOLUME OF DISTRIBUTION (Vd)

The volume of distribution for a drug or the "apparent volume of distribution," does not necessarily refer to any real volume (1,43). It is simply the size of a compartment necessary to account for the total amount of drug in the body if it were present throughout the body in the same concentration found in the plasma. See Fig. 6A. The equation for the volume of distribution is expressed as follows:

$$Vd = \frac{Ab}{Cp} \qquad \text{(Eq. 9)}$$

where Vd is the apparent volume of distribution, Ab is the total amount of drug in the body, and Cp is the plasma concentration of drug.

Apparent volumes of distribution which are larger than the plasma compartment (> 3L) only indicate that the drug is also present in tissues or fluids outside that compartment. The actual sites of distribution cannot be determined from this value.

The apparent volume of distribution is a function of the lipid versus water solubilities and of the plasma and tissue protein

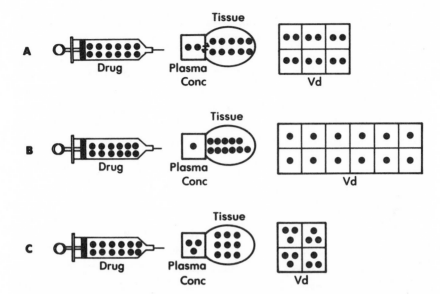

Fig. 6. Volume of Distribution. (A) The administration of a given amount of drug into the body produces a specific plasma concentration. The apparent volume of distribution which accounts for the total dose administered based upon the observed plasma concentration is depicted. (B) Any factor which decreases the plasma concentration, such as decreased plasma protein binding, will increase the apparent volume of distribution. (C) Conversely, any factor which increases the plasma concentration, such as decreased tissue binding, will decrease the apparent volume of distribution.

binding properties of the drug. Factors which tend to keep the drug in the plasma or increase Cp, such as low lipid solubility, increased plasma protein binding, or decreased tissue binding, *reduce* the apparent volume of distribution. It follows then that factors which decrease Cp, such as decreased plasma protein binding, increased tissue binding, and increased lipid solubility, *increase* the apparent volume of distribution.

Loading Dose

Since the volume of distribution is the factor which accounts for all of the drug in the body, it can be used to estimate the loading dose necessary to rapidly achieve a desired plasma concentration:

$$\text{Loading Dose} = \frac{(Vd)(Cp)}{(S)(F)} \qquad \text{(Eq. 10)}$$

where Vd is the volume of distribution, Cp is the desired plasma level and (S)(F) represents the fraction of the dose administered that will reach the systemic circulation (see Fig. 7). For example, if one wished to calculate an oral loading dose of digoxin for a 70 kg man which would produce a plasma concentration of 1.5 ng/ml (mcg/L), Eq. 10 would be used. If S is assumed to be 1.0, F to be 0.62, and the volume of distribution to be 7.3 L/kg (31,42), the loading dose would be 1236 mcg or 1.236 mg based upon the following calculation:

$$\frac{(7.3 \text{ L/kg})(70 \text{ kg})(1.5 \text{ mcg/L})}{(1.0)(0.62)} = 1236 \text{ mcg or } 1.236 \text{ mg}$$

A reasonable approximation of this dose would be 1.25 mg given orally as tablets. The usual clinical approach would be to give the loading dose in divided doses (0.25–0.5 mg per dose) every six hours and observe the patient before each successive dose is administered. In addition, clinicians frequently use a bioavailability factor greater than 0.62 (e.g., 0.7 or 0.75) to guard against "overshooting" the desired level.

Equation 10 can also be used to estimate the loading dose required to achieve a higher plasma concentration when some initial concentration is already present. See Fig. 8. This new formula is derived by replacing the Cp in Eq. 10 by an expression which represents the increment in plasma concentration which is desired.

$$\textbf{Loading Dose} = \frac{(\textbf{Vd})(\textbf{Cp desired} - \textbf{Cp initial})}{(\textbf{S})(\textbf{F})} \qquad \text{(Eq. 11)}$$

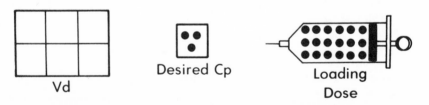

Vd   Desired Cp   Loading Dose

Fig. 7. Loading Dose. The volume of distribution is the major determinant of the loading dose. If the Vd for a drug is known and one wishes to achieve a specific plasma concentration, the loading dose which will produce that concentration is easily calculated. See Eq. 10.

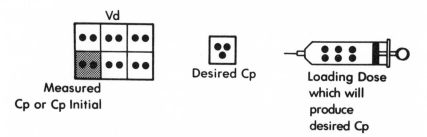

Fig. 8. Loading Dose to Produce an Increment in Plasma Level. If the Vd and plasma concentration for a drug are known and one wishes to achieve a higher plasma concentration, the loading dose which will produce that increment can be calculated. See Eq. 11.

For example, if the previous patient had a digoxin level of 0.5 mcg/L and the desired concentration was 1.5 mcg/L, the loading dose would have been:

$$\frac{(7.3 \text{ L/kg})(70 \text{ kg})(1.5 \text{ mcg/L} - 0.5 \text{ mcg/L})}{(1.0)(0.62)} = 824 \text{ mcg or } 0.824 \text{ mg}$$

A reasonable total loading dose in this case would be about 0.75 mg.

Factors Which Alter Vd and Loading Dose

In analyzing Eq. 10, it becomes clear that any factor which alters the volume of distribution will theoretically influence the loading dose which should be administered. *Decreased tissue binding* of drugs in uremic patients is a common cause of a reduced apparent volume of distribution for several agents (28). See Fig. 6C. Decreased tissue binding will increase the Cp by allowing more of the drug to remain in the plasma. Therefore, if the desired plasma level remains unchanged, a smaller loading dose will be required. Digoxin is an example of a drug whose loading dose must be altered in uremic patients. This is discussed in Part Two in the Digoxin chapter.

Decreased plasma protein binding, on the other hand, tends to increase the apparent volume of distribution because more drug is available for tissue binding sites. See Fig. 6B. However, as discussed in the section on Desired Plasma Concentration, decreased plasma protein binding also increases the fraction of free or active drug so that the desired Cp which produces a given therapeutic response decreases. To summarize, diminished plasma protein binding increases Vd and decreases Cp in Eq. 10 so that there is generally no net effect on the loading dose. This is based upon the assumption that the majority of drug in the body is actually outside the plasma compartment and the amount of drug bound to plasma protein comprises only a small percentage of the total amount in the body.

This principle is illustrated by the pharmacokinetic behavior of phenytoin in uremic patients. Plasma phenytoin levels in uremic patients are one-half of those observed in normal patients, following a single intravenous dose. However, because the free fraction (alpha) increases from 0.12 to 0.25, the lower plasma levels produce the same free or pharmacologically active concentration. Furthermore, because the volume of distribution increases by approximately two-fold (0.65 L/kg to 1.44 L/kg), the loading dose of phenytoin which produces the same therapeutic effect would be the same for both the uremic and non-uremic patients (40). This assumes there is no change in bioavailability:

$$(2 \times \text{Vd})(\tfrac{1}{2} \times \text{Cp desired}) = \text{No change in LD} \qquad \text{(Eq. 10)}$$

Two Compartment Models

If one thinks of the body as a single compartment, pharmacokinetic calculations are relatively simple. However, there are some situations when it is more appropriate to consider the body as two, and occasionally more than two compartments. The first compartment can be thought of as a rapidly equilibrating volume, *usually* made up of blood and those organs or tissues which have high blood-flow. This first compartment has a volume referred to as Vi or initial volume. The second compartment requires a somewhat longer time period to equilibrate with the drug. This volume is referred to as Vt or tissue volume (43). The half-time of the distribution phase is referred to as the alpha (α) half-life, and the half-time of drug elimination from the body is referred to as the beta (β) half-life. The sum of

Vi and Vt is the apparent volume of distribution (Vd). Drugs are assumed to enter into and be eliminated from Vi. See Fig. 9.

Because some time is required for a drug to distribute into Vt, a rapidly administered loading dose calculated on the basis Vd (Vi + Vt) would result in an initial Cp larger than predicted because of the smaller initial volume of distribution (Vi). The consequences of such an inaccurate prediction depend on whether the target organ behaves as though it were located in Vi or Vt. Drugs such as lidocaine, quinidine, and procainamide exert therapeutic and toxic effects on target organs which behave as though they were located in Vi. In these instances, the concentration of drug in the target organs could be much higher than expected and produce toxicity if appropriate adjustments in the administration of the loading dose are not made. This problem can be circumvented by calculating the total loading dose based on Vd. Then, the loading dose should be administered at a rate slow enough to allow for drug distribution into Vt, or the total loading dose should be given in sufficiently small increments so that the Cp in Vi does not exceed some predetermined critical concentration (22,37).

When the drug's target organ is in the second or tissue compartment Vt (e.g., digoxin), the rather high Cp which may be observed prior to distribution is not dangerous. Plasma concentrations which are obtained before distribution is complete will not reflect the tissue concentration at equilibrium, and, therefore, these plasma samples cannot be used to predict therapeutic or toxic effects of these drugs (51,53). For example, clinicians usually wait several hours after an intravenous loading dose before evaluating the effect of digoxin. This delay allows the digoxin to distribute to the site of action (myocardium) so that the full therapeutic or toxic effects of a dose can be observed. See Digoxin chapter, Fig. 1.

The problem of slow drug distribution into tissue is most significant when the drug is given by the intravenous route. It is generally not a problem when a drug is given orally because the rate of absorption is usually slower than the rate of distribution from Vi into Vt. However, digoxin is an exception to this rule. Even when digoxin is given orally, a minimum of six hours is required for complete absorption and distribution. Digoxin plasma samples obtained less than six hours after an oral dose are of questionable value because the plasma concentration will initially be elevated (distribution into Vt is still taking place) and the pharmacologic response will be much less than the plasma concentration would indicate.

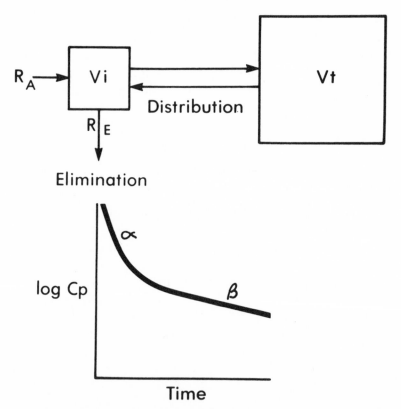

Fig. 9. Two Compartment Model. Volumes of distribution for a two-compartment model. Vi is the initial volume of distribution. Note that drug administration and elimination (R_E) are assumed to occur in Vi. The lower graph shows how a drug administered into Vi follows a biphasic decay pattern. The initial decay half-life ($\alpha t\frac{1}{2}$) is usually due to drug being distributed into Vt. The second decay half-life ($\beta t\frac{1}{2}$) is usually due to drug being eliminated from the body.

CLEARANCE (Cl)

The rapid achievement of a desired drug concentration in the plasma by administration of a loading dose has been presented. To maintain that desired drug concentration, the drug must be replaced at a rate equal to its loss. The pharmacokinetic parameter which accounts for drug loss from the body is clearance. At steady state, the rate of drug administration (R_A) and rate of drug elimination (R_E) must be equal (also see next section on Elimination Rate Constant).

$$R_A = R_E \qquad \text{(Eq. 12)}$$

Clearance (Cl) can best be thought of as the proportionality constant that makes the average steady state plasma level of drug equal to the rate of drug administration (R_A):

$$R_A = (Cl)(Cpss\ ave) \qquad \text{(Eq. 13)}$$

where R_A is $(S)(F)(Dose/\tau)$ (see Eq. 4) and Cpss ave is the average steady state drug concentration. Clearance can also be thought of as the intrinsic ability of the body or its organs of elimination (usually the kidneys and the liver) to remove drug from the blood or plasma. Clearance is expressed as a volume per unit of time. It is important to emphasize that clearance is *not* an indicator of *how much* drug is being removed; it only represents the theoretical volume of blood or plasma which is completely cleared of drug in a given period of time. The *amount* of drug removed depends on the plasma concentration of drug as well as the clearance. See Fig. 10.

If an average steady state plasma concentration and rate of drug administration are known, the clearance can be calculated by rearranging Eq. 13:

$$Cl = \frac{(S)(F)(Dose/\tau)}{Cpss\ ave} \qquad \text{(Eq. 14)}$$

For example, if intravenous lidocaine is infused continually at a rate of 2 mg/min and if the concentration of lidocaine at steady state is 3 mg/L, the calculated lidocaine clearance using Eq. 14 would be 0.667 L/min:

$$\frac{(1.0)(1.0)(2 \text{ mg/min})}{3 \text{ mg/L}} = 0.667 \text{ L/min}$$

"F" is considered to be 1.0 because the drug is being administered intravenously. "S" is also assumed to be 1.0 because the hydrochloride salt represents only a small fraction of the total molecular weight for lidocaine and correction is unnecessary.

STEADY STATE

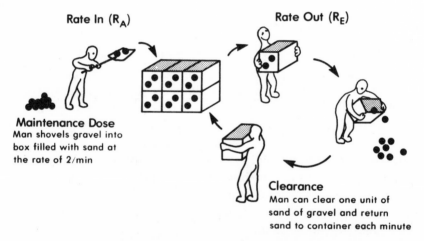

Fig. 10. Steady State, Maintenance Dose, Clearance, Elimination Rate Constant.
At steady state the rate of drug administration (R_A) is equal to the rate of drug elimination (R_E) and the concentration of drug remains constant. In this example, the man on the left is able to shovel gravel or "drug" into a container of sand at the rate of 2/minute. The man on the right is able to remove one unit of sand with its gravel or "drug" from the container, dump the gravel, and return the sand to the container each minute. The *amount* of gravel or drug removed per unit of time (rate of elimination) will be determined by the concentration of gravel per unit as well as the clearance (volume of sand cleared of gravel). The elimination rate constant (Kd) can be thought of as the fraction of the total volume cleared per unit of time. In this case Kd would be equal to ⅙ or 0.17 min⁻¹.

Maintenance Dose

If an estimate for clearance is obtained from the literature, the clearance formula (Eq. 14) can be rearranged slightly and used to calculate the rate of administration or maintenance dose which will produce a desired average plasma concentration at steady state:

$$\text{Maintenance Dose} = \frac{(Cl)(Cpss\ ave)(\tau)}{(S)(F)} \qquad \text{(Eq. 15)}$$

For example, using the estimate for theophylline clearance of 2.8 L/hr which is reported in the literature, one could determine the rate of intravenous administration for aminophylline which would produce a given steady state plasma theophylline concentration of 15 mg/L. This is illustrated below:

$$\frac{(2.8\ \text{L/hr})(15\ \text{mg/L})(1\ \text{hr})}{(0.8)(1.0)} = 52.5\ \text{mg/hr}$$

Since τ was one hour, the rate of administration would be 52.5 mg/hr. If the aminophylline were to be given every six hours, the dose would be 315 mg or six times the hourly administration rate.

Factors Which Alter Clearance (See Table 2)

Body Surface Area (BSA). Most literature values for clearance are expressed as volume/time/kg or as volume/time/70 kg. There is some evidence, however, that drug clearance is best adjusted on the basis of body surface area rather than on weight (6,16,17,50). Body surface area can be calculated using Eq. 16 or it can be obtained from various charts and nomograms (44,46). See Appendix I.

$$\text{BSA in m}^2 = \left(\frac{\text{Patient's weight in kg}}{70\ \text{kg}} \right)^{0.73} (1.73\ \text{m}^2) \qquad \text{(Eq. 16)}$$

The following formulas can be used to adjust the clearance values reported in the literature for specific patients:

Table 2
FACTORS WHICH ALTER CLEARANCE

Body Weight
Body Surface Area
Plasma Protein Binding
High Extraction Ratio
Renal Function
Hepatic Function
Decreased Cardiac Output

$$\text{Patient's Cl} = (\text{Literature Cl/70 kg}) \left(\frac{\text{Patient's BSA}}{1.73 \text{ m}^2} \right) \qquad \text{(Eq. 17)}$$

$$\text{Patient's Cl} = (\text{Literature Cl/70 kg}) \left(\frac{\text{Patient's wt in kg}}{70 \text{ kg}} \right) \qquad \text{(Eq. 18)}$$

$$\text{Patient's Cl} = (\text{Literature Cl/kg})(\text{Patient's wt in kg}) \qquad \text{(Eq. 19)}$$

Equations 18 and 19 adjust clearance in proportion to weight, whereas Eq. 17 adjusts the clearance in proportion to body surface area. If the patient's weight is reasonably close to 70 kg (BSA = 1.73 m²), the corrected clearance will be approximately the same using all three approaches.

Plasma Protein Binding. For highly protein-bound drugs, diminished plasma protein binding is associated with a decrease in reported steady state plasma drug concentration (total of bound plus free drug) for any given dose which is administered. See Fig. 5 and the discussion of binding affinity in the section on Desired Plasma Concentration. By examination of Eq. 14, it can be seen that a decrease in the denominator, Cpss ave, results in an increase in the calculated clearance.

$$\text{Cl} = \frac{(\text{S})(\text{F})(\text{Dose/}\tau)}{\text{Cpss ave}} \qquad \text{(Eq. 14)}$$

It would be misleading, however, to assume that because the calculated clearance is increased that the *amount* eliminated per unit of time has doubled. This is because Eq. 14 assumes that when Cpss ave (total of bound plus free drug) changes, there is a proportionate change in the free drug concentration which is available for metabolism and renal elimination. In actuality, the free or unbound fraction of drug in the plasma (61) generally increases with diminished plasma protein binding and the *amount* of free drug eliminated per unit of time remains unchanged. This should be apparent if one considers that at steady state the amount of drug administered per unit of time (R_A) must equal the amount eliminated per unit of time (R_E). If R_A has not changed, R_E must remain the same. To summarize, when the same daily dose of a drug is given in the presence of diminished protein binding, an amount equal to that dose will be eliminated from the body each day at steady state despite a diminished steady state plasma concentration and increase in the calculated clearance. Furthermore, because this lower plasma concentration is associated with an increased fraction of free drug, the pharmacologic effect achieved will be similar to that produced by the higher serum concentration observed in the presence of normal protein binding. This example re-emphasizes the principle that clearance alone is not a good indicator of the *amount* of drug eliminated per unit of time (R_E). See Figs. 11 and 12.

STEADY STATE

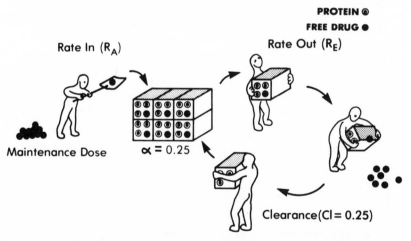

Fig. 11. Clearance of a Highly Protein Bound Drug with a Low Extraction Ratio. Note that it is the free drug fraction (α) that is available for clearance. Protein-bound drug is returned to the container so that the actual volume cleared of drug is ¼ of the volume removed by the man on the right each minute. Compare with Fig. 10.

STEADY STATE

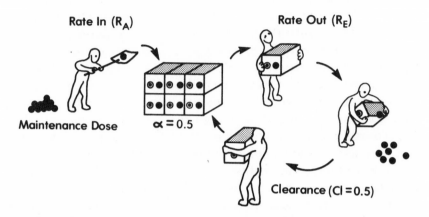

Rate In (R$_A$)   Rate Out (R$_E$)

Maintenance Dose $\alpha = 0.5$

Clearance (Cl = 0.5)

Fig. 12. **Effect of Diminished Protein Binding on Clearance of a Highly Protein Bound Drug Which Has a Low Extraction Ratio.** Compare this figure with Fig. 11. Note that the plasma concentration of drug has decreased but that the free concentration remains the same (α is increased). See Fig. 4. The volume actually cleared of drug has increased as compared to that cleared in Fig. 11 even though the amount of drug cleared per unit of time has remained unchanged. This illustrates the principle that the amount of a highly protein bound drug cleared per unit of time (R$_E$) remains the same if the increase in clearance is proportional to the increase in fraction free when protein binding is decreased.

This principle is illustrated by comparing the calculated clearances at steady state for a uremic and nonuremic patient, both of whom are receiving 300 mg of phenytoin daily. As noted previously, (see section on Desired Plasma Concentration, discussion of binding affinity), the steady state plasma phenytoin concentration in the uremic individual receiving 300 mg daily will be lower ($\approx$ 4 mg/L) than that of the nonuremic patient ($\approx$ 10 mg/L) because of decreased protein binding. However, even with this disparity in measured plasma concentrations, the concentration of free or active drug will be approximately the same for both patients because the alpha or fraction free is equal to 0.25 in the uremic and 0.1 in the non-uremic individual. Consequently, even though the calculated clearance for the uremic patient is higher than the nonuremic patient (75 L/day vs 30 L/day), the amount of drug cleared per day (300 mg) is the same. To summarize, when protein binding is decreased, the increase in calculated clearance is generally directly proportional to the change in alpha. Although the calculated clearance may be used to estimate a maintenance dose, it is the selection of a plasma level which will produce the desired pharmacologic effect which is most critical to the determination of a therapeutically correct maintenance dose.

Extraction Ratio. The direct proportionality between calculated clearance and alpha is not observed for drugs which are metabolized or excreted so efficiently that some (perhaps all) of the drug bound to plasma protein is removed as it passes through the eliminating organ (7,19). In this situation the plasma protein acts as a "transport system" for the drug, carrying it to the eliminating organs, and the clearance becomes dependent upon the blood or plasma flow to the eliminating organ. To determine whether the clearance for a drug is primarily dependent upon blood flow or protein binding, its extraction ratio can be estimated and compared to its alpha value.

The extraction ratio is the fraction of the drug presented to the eliminating organ which is cleared after a single pass through that organ. It can be estimated by dividing the blood or plasma clearance of a drug by the blood or plasma flow to the eliminating organ. If the extraction ratio exceeds alpha, then the plasma proteins are acting as a transport system and clearance will not increase proportionately to a change in alpha. If, however, the extraction ratio is less than alpha, it is probable that clearance will appear to increase by the same proportion that alpha changes. This approach does not take into account other factors which may affect clearance such as the binding to or the elimination from red blood cells or changes in metabolic function.

Renal and Hepatic Function; Cardiac Output. Drug elimination or clearance occurs by two major routes: as unchanged drug through the kidney (renal clearance) and by metabolism in the liver (metabolic clearance). These two routes are assumed to be independent of one another and additive (43).

$$Cl_t = Cl_m + Cl_r \qquad \text{(Eq. 20)}$$

where Cl_t is total clearance, Cl_m is metabolic clearance or the fraction cleared by metabolism, and Cl_r is renal clearance or the fraction cleared by the renal route. Since the kidneys and liver function independently, it is assumed that a change in one does not affect the other. Thus, Cl_t can be estimated in the presence of renal or hepatic failure or both. If the metabolic and renal clearances for a drug are known, the clearance for the affected route can be reduced proportionately before the Cl_t is calculated. Since metabolic function is difficult to quantitate, this approach is most often used when there is decreased renal function:

$$Cl_{adjusted} = Cl_m + (Cl_r \times \text{Fraction of Normal Renal Function Remaining}) \qquad \text{(Eq. 21)}$$

The value of a clearance which has been adjusted for renal function is that it can be used to estimate the maintenance dose for a patient in renal failure. See Eq. 15. However, it is only valid to use the adjusted clearance if the drug's metabolites are inactive and the metabolic clearance is unaffected by renal failure.

A decrease in the function of an organ of elimination is most significant when that organ serves as the primary route of drug elimination. However, as the major elimination pathway becomes increasingly compromised, the "minor" pathway becomes more significant because it assumes a greater portion of the total clearance. For example, a drug which is usually 67% eliminated by the renal route and 33% by the metabolic route will be 100% metabolized in the event of complete renal failure; the total clearance, however, will only be one-third of the normal value.

Most pharmacokinetic adjustments for drug elimination are based upon renal function because hepatic function is usually more difficult to quantitate. Hepatic function can be evaluated using the prothrombin time, serum albumin and serum bilirubin concentrations. Unfortunately, each of these laboratory tests is affected by variables other than altered hepatic function. For example, the serum albumin may be low due to decreased protein intake, increased renal or gastrointestinal loss, as well as to decreased hepatic function. Although liver function tests

NON STEADY STATE

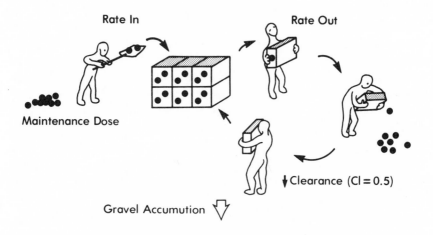

Rate In

Maintenance Dose

Rate Out

↓Clearance (Cl = 0.5)

Gravel Accumution ▽

NEW STEADY STATE

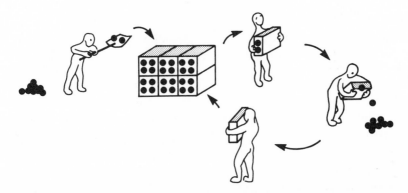

Fig. 13. Effect of Changes in Clearance on Steady State Serum Concentrations.
Compare this figure with Fig. 10. In the illustration above, the maintenance
dose or amount of gravel added to the container per unit of time remains the
same; however, the volume of sand cleared of gravel (clearance) has been
halved. Initially, the amount of gravel or "drug" cleared per unit of time is less
than the maintenance dose. Because of this, the concentration of gravel increases until a new steady state is reached. At this point the rate at which
gravel is added to the container again equals the rate at which gravel is
eliminated from the container. If clearance had increased, the concentration of
gravel would have decreased until the amount removed per unit of time (R_E)
again equaled the rate of administration (R_A).

31

do not provide quantitative data, pharmacokinetic adjustments must still consider liver function because of the importance of this route of elimination.

It has recently become apparent that cardiac output affects drug metabolism. Hepatic or metabolic clearances for some drugs can be decreased by 25 to 50% in patients with congestive heart failure. For example, the metabolic clearance of theophylline (4) and digoxin (6) appears to be reduced by about one-half of normal in patients with congestive heart failure. This finding is interesting since the metabolic clearance for both of these drugs is much less than the hepatic blood or plasma flow (low extraction ratio), and it would not have been predicted that their clearances would have been influenced by cardiac output or hepatic blood flow to this extent. The decreased cardiac output and resultant hepatic congestion must, in some way, decrease the intrinsic metabolic capacity of the liver. The effect of diminished clearance on plasma drug concentrations is illustrated in Fig. 13 (compare with Fig. 10).

ELIMINATION RATE CONSTANT (Kd) AND HALF-LIFE (t½)

In the preceding sections, a method of drug dosing which utilized a loading dose followed by a maintenance dose was presented. However, loading doses are not used in many clinical situations; instead, maintenance doses of a drug are simply initiated. In these instances, it is often desirable to predict how drug plasma levels will change with time. For drugs which are eliminated by first-order kinetics, these predictions are based upon the elimination rate constant (Kd).

First-Order Kinetics

First-order elimination kinetics refers to the process whereby the *amount* or concentration of drug in the body diminishes logarithmically over time (see Fig. 14).

The rate of elimination (R_E) is proportional to the drug concentration; therefore the amount removed per unit of time (R_E) will vary proportionately with drug concentration, but the *fraction or percentage* of the total amount of drug present in the

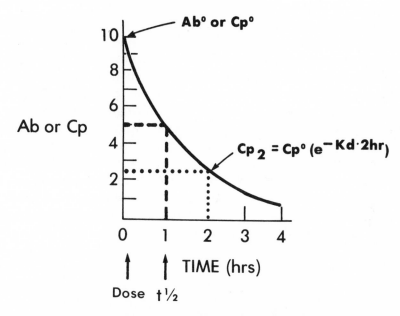

Fig. 14. First-Order Elimination. The amount or concentration of drug diminishes logarithmically over time. The initial amount or plasma concentration produced by a loading dose is Ab^0 or Cp^0. The half-life ($t\frac{1}{2}$) is the time required to eliminate one-half of the drug. The concentration at the end of a given time interval (in this example, 2 hours) is equal to the initial concentration times the fraction of drug remaining at the end of that time interval ($e^{-Kd\cdot 2\,hr}$). Note that the amount or concentration of drug lost in each time interval of 1 hour diminishes over time ($5 \longrightarrow 2.5 \longrightarrow 1.25$); however, the fraction of drug which is lost each unit of time (0.5) remains constant. For example, over the first hour, one-half of the total amount of drug in the body (10) was lost (5). In the next time interval (1–2 hrs), one-half of the amount of drug which remained (5) was lost (2.5).

body (Ab) which is removed at any instant in time will remain constant and independent of dose. That fraction or percentage is expressed by the Elimination Rate Constant, Kd. The equation which describes first-order elimination of a drug from the body is:

$$Ab = (Ab^0)(e^{-Kdt}) \quad \text{or}$$

$$Cp = (Cp^0)(e^{-Kdt}) \tag{Eq. 22}$$

where Ab^0 and Ab represent the total amount of drug in the body at the beginning and end of the time interval t, and e^{-Kdt}

is the fraction of Ab remaining at time t. Cp^0 and Cp are the plasma concentrations at the beginning and end of the time interval respectively. Since the drug concentration diminishes logarithmically, a graphic plot of the natural logarithm of the plasma level versus time yields a straight line (see Fig. 15).

This type of graphical analysis of declining plasma drug concentrations is often used to determine if a drug is eliminated by a first-order process. Another important characteristic of first-order elimination is that both clearance and volume of distribution remain constant and do not vary with dose. This means that adjustments of drug concentrations can be made by altering the drug dosage in proportion to the desired change in concentration. See Fig. 16.

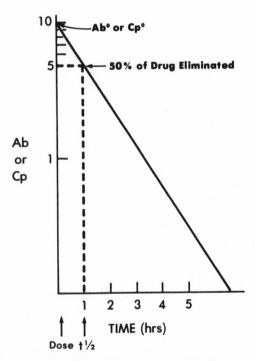

Fig. 15. **First-Order Elimination.** A graph of the log of Ab or Cp versus time yields a straight line. The half-life is the time required for Ab or Cp to decline to one-half the original value.

NON STEADY STATE

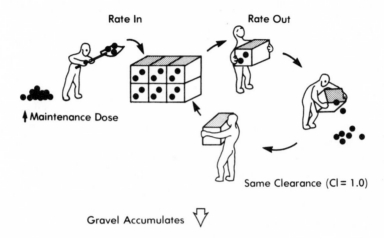

Rate In   Rate Out

↟ Maintenance Dose

Same Clearance (Cl = 1.0)

Gravel Accumulates ▽

NEW STEADY STATE

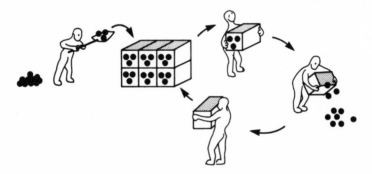

Fig. 16. **Effect of Changes in Maintenance Dose on Steady State Plasma Concentrations.** Compare this figure with Fig. 10. In the illustration above, the clearance or volume of sand cleared of gravel remains the same; however, the maintenance dose or the amount of gravel added to the container per unit of time has been increased from 2/minute to 3/minute. Because of this, the concentration of gravel or "drug" increases until a new steady state is reached. At this point, the rate at which gravel is added to the container again equals the rate at which gravel is eliminated from the container. Had the maintenance dose decreased, the concentration of gravel would have gradually decreased until a new steady state had been achieved.

Elimination Rate Constant (Kd)

The elimination rate constant, Kd, is the fraction or percentage of the total amount of drug in the body removed per unit of time and it is a function of clearance and volume of distribution:

$$Kd = \frac{Cl}{Vd} \qquad \text{(Eq. 23)}$$

As Eq. 23 demonstrates, Kd can also be thought of as the fraction of the volume of distribution which will be effectively cleared of drug per unit of time. See Fig. 10. For example, a drug with a clearance of 10 L/day and a Vd of 100 L would have an elimination rate constant of 0.1 days^{-1}.

Since the drug elimination rate constant is the slope of the ln Cp vs time plot, it can be calculated for a specific patient using two plasma concentrations measured during the decay or elimination phase (i.e., between doses or following a single dose) using Eq. 24:

$$Kd = \frac{\ln\left(\frac{Cp_1}{Cp_2}\right)}{t} \qquad \text{(Eq. 24)}$$

where Cp_1 is the first or higher plasma concentration and Cp_2 is the second or lower plasma concentration, and t is the time interval between the plasma samples. For example, if Cp_1 was 5 mg/L and Cp_2 was 2 mg/L, with the time interval between the samples being 8 hours, the elimination rate constant (Kd) would be 0.115 hr^{-1}:

$$Kd = \frac{\ln\left(\frac{5 \text{ mg/L}}{2 \text{ mg/L}}\right)}{8 \text{ hrs}} = 0.115 \text{ hr}^{-1}$$

For an accurate estimate of Kd, the time which has elapsed between samples should span at least one half-life (see next section on Half-life). Although Kd is dependent upon the volume of distribution and clearance (not vice versa as discussed later), some authors have suggested that Kd be adjusted for renal failure in a manner similar to that discussed for clearance, and that the adjusted Kd be used to estimate a clearance value in renal failure using Eq. 26 (27,52). See section on Clearance: Factors Which Alter Clearance, and Eq. 21.

$$Kd_{adjusted} = K_{metabolic} + \left(K_{renal} \times \begin{array}{l} \textbf{Fraction of Normal} \\ \textbf{Renal Function} \\ \textbf{Remaining} \end{array} \right) \qquad \text{(Eq. 25)}$$

$$Cl_{adjusted} = (Kd_{adjusted})(Vd_{normal}) \qquad \text{(Eq. 26)}$$

This adjusted clearance is then used to calculate a maintenance dose for the patient in renal failure using Eq. 15:

$$\text{Maintenance Dose} = \frac{(Cl)(Cpss\ ave)(\tau)}{(S)(F)} \qquad \text{(Eq. 15)}$$

This method is based on the assumption that changes in clearance are proportional to changes in Kd if the volume of distribution does not change in renal failure. However, this is often not the case. As noted previously in the discussion of Vd, protein binding changes which occur in renal failure also produce changes in the volume of distribution (see Fig. 6). Nevertheless, one may occasionally have to resort to this indirect method of determining clearance because presently elimination rate constants for drugs are more readily available in the literature than are clearance values. While the adjusted Kd calculated by this approach may be satisfactorily used to estimate an adjusted clearance in renal failure, it *cannot* be reliably used to estimate the half-life of a drug in a patient with renal failure if the Vd is altered (33,52). If Vd is altered in renal failure and if the indirect method of determining clearance is being utilized, the normal value for Vd must still be used in Eq. 26 because Kd was adjusted on the assumption that Vd had *not* changed in renal failure.

Half-life (t½)

The elimination rate constant is often expressed as the drug's half-life, which may be more conveniently applied to the clinical setting. The half-life (t½) of a drug is the amount of time required for the total amount of drug in the body or the plasma drug concentration to decrease by one-half. See Fig. 15. It is some-times referred to as the $\beta t\frac{1}{2}$ to distinguish it from the half-life for distribution ($\alpha t\frac{1}{2}$) in a two compartment model and it is a function of the elimination rate constant, Kd:

$$t\frac{1}{2} = \frac{0.693}{Kd} \qquad \text{(Eq. 27)}$$

If the Kd used in Eq. 27 is derived from plasma concentrations obtained during the decay phase (See discussion of Eq. 24), then the time interval in which the samples are drawn should span at least one half-life. Shorter time periods can be used, but small errors in the assayed concentrations can alter the calculated half-life considerably. This rule makes it impractical to obtain peak and trough levels within a dosing interval to determine the half-life because the dosing interval is frequently equal to or shorter than the usual half-life for most drugs (e.g., theophylline, quinidine, procainamide, digoxin, phenobarbital).

If the volume of distribution and clearance for a drug are known, it is more valid and practical to estimate half-life using Eq. 28 below. Because half-life is a function of Kd, it too is dependent upon and determined by Cl and Vd. This relationship is illustrated by Eq. 28 which was obtained by substituting Eq. 23 into Eq. 27:

$$t\frac{1}{2} = \frac{(0.693)(Vd)}{Cl} \qquad \text{(Eq. 28)}$$

The importance of emphasizing the dependence of $t\frac{1}{2}$ or Kd on these two parameters is that in a variety of clinical circumstances, the volume of distribution and clearance for a drug may change *independently* of one another and thus affect the half-life or elimination constant in the same or opposite directions.

Another caution is appropriate at this point. It is a common misconception that because Eq. 23 can be rearranged to:

$$Cl = (Kd)(Vd) \qquad \text{(Eq. 29)}$$

that clearance is determined by Kd (or $t\frac{1}{2}$) and Vd; however, this is incorrect. Instead, Kd and $t\frac{1}{2}$ are dependent upon clearance and the volume of distribution; it is therefore invalid to make any assumptions about the Vd or clearance of a drug based solely upon knowledge of its half-life. For example, if the half-life of a drug is prolonged, the clearance may be increased, decreased, or the same depending upon corresponding changes in the volume of distribution.

Clinical Application of Kd and Half-Life (See Table 3)

Time to Reach Steady State. Half-life is an important variable to consider when answering questions concerning time such as "How long will it take a patient to reach steady state on a constant dosage regimen?" or "How long will it take the patient to reach steady state if the dosage regimen is changed?" When drugs are given chronically, they accumulate in the body until the amount administered in a given time period (maintenance dose) is equal to the amount eliminated in that same period. When this occurs, drug concentrations in the plasma will plateau and the patient will be at "steady state." See Figs. 10 and 11. The time required for a drug to reach steady state levels is determined by its half-life. It takes one half-life to reach 50%, two half-lives to reach 75%, three half-lives to reach 87.5%, and four half-lives to reach 93.75% of steady state. *In most clinical situations, it is sufficient to wait three to four half-lives before the attainment of steady state can effectively be assumed.* See Fig. 17.

Table 3
CLINICAL APPLICATION OF THE ELIMINATION RATE CONSTANT (Kd)
AND HALF-LIFE (t½)

1. Estimation of the time to reach steady state plasma concentrations after initiation of a maintenance dose or after a change in the maintenance dose.

2. Estimation of the time required to eliminate all or a portion of the drug from the body once it is discontinued.

3. Prediction of non-steady state plasma levels following the initiation of an infusion.

4. Prediction of a steady state plasma level from a non-steady state plasma level obtained at a specific time following the initiation of an infusion.

5. Given the degree of fluctuation in plasma concentration desired within a dosing interval, determine that interval.

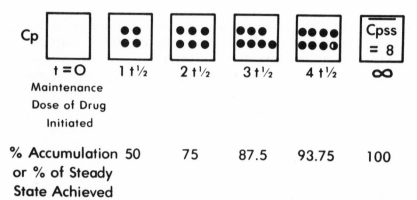

Cp

t = O
Maintenance
Dose of Drug
Initiated

1 t½   2 t½   3 t½   4 t½   ∞

Cpss = 8

% Accumulation 50   75   87.5   93.75   100
or % of Steady
State Achieved

Fig. 17. **First-Order Accumulation.** When a maintenance dose is initiated, it takes 4 or more half-lives to reach steady state plasma drug levels. This example assumes that the maintenance dose administered will produce an average steady state level (Cpss ave or C̄pss) of 8.

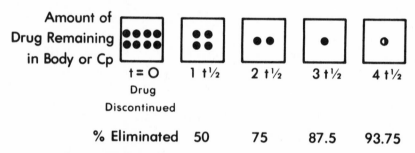

Amount of
Drug Remaining
in Body or Cp

t = O
Drug
Discontinued

1 t½   2 t½   3 t½   4 t½

% Eliminated   50   75   87.5   93.75

Fig. 18. **First-Order Elimination. Amount of Drug Remaining in the Body After One to Four Half-lives Have Passed.** Note that the amount of drug eliminated per unit of time diminishes over time, but that the fraction eliminated in each time interval (In this case, 0.5) remains the same.

Time for Drug Elimination. Conversely, the half-life can also be used to determine how long it will take to effectively eliminate all of the drug from the body once it has been discontinued. It takes one half-life to eliminate 50%, two half-lives to eliminate 75%, three half-lives to eliminate 87.5%, and four half-lives to eliminate 93.75% of the total amount of drug in the body. Again, in *most* clinical situations it is sufficient to wait .hree to four half-lives before it can be assumed that all of the drug has been effectively eliminated. See Fig. 18.

Since the concept of half-life does not answer the question "how much?", the actual magnitude of the plasma levels which are ultimately attained from a given dosage regimen is not considered in the principle stated above.

Prediction of Plasma Levels Following Initiation of an Infusion. Often, when drugs are given by constant infusion, it is useful to predict the plasma concentrations which will be achieved at a specific period of time prior to steady state. See Fig. 23. The rate at which a drug approaches steady state is governed by the elimination rate constant; therefore, this parameter can be used to calculate the fraction of steady state which is achieved any time after the initiation of the infusion (t_1):

$$\text{Fraction of Steady State Achieved at } t_1 = (1 - e^{-Kdt_1}) \qquad \text{(Eq. 30)}$$

The average plasma concentration at steady state (Cpss ave) can be calculated by rearranging the clearance formula (Eq. 14):

$$Cl = \frac{(S)(F)(Dose/\tau)}{Cpss\ ave} \qquad \text{(Eq. 14)}$$

$$Cpss\ ave = \frac{(S)(F)(Dose/\tau)}{Cl} \qquad \text{(Eq. 31)}$$

and the plasma level which can be expected at a specific time after initiation of the infusion (t_1) can be calculated by multiplying the average steady state concentration by the fraction of steady state achieved at t_1.

$$\text{Plasma Conc. at } t_1 = (\text{Cpss ave})\left(\begin{array}{c}\text{Fraction of Steady State}\\ \text{Achieved at } t_1\end{array}\right)$$

$$\begin{array}{l}\text{Fraction of Steady State}\\ \text{Achieved at } t_1\end{array} = (1 - e^{-Kdt_1}) \qquad \text{(Eq. 30)}$$

Plasma Conc. at t_1 = (Cpss ave)$(1 - e^{-Kdt_1})$

$$= \frac{\textbf{(S)(F)(Dose/}\tau\textbf{)}}{\textbf{Cl}} \times (1 - e^{-Kdt_1}) \qquad \textbf{(Eq. 32)}$$

All of the time units used in Eq. 32 (τ, Cl, t_1) should be the same. Note that as t_1 approaches four or more half-lives, the fraction of steady state achieved approaches one.

Conversely, if one has a plasma concentration from a sample which was drawn prior to steady state, the approximate steady state concentration which will be achieved can be estimated through rearrangement of Eq. 32:

$$\textbf{Cpss ave} = \frac{\textbf{Plasma Concentration at } t_1}{(1 - e^{-Kdt_1})} \qquad \textbf{(Eq. 33)}$$

If the predicted steady state concentration is too high, side effects or toxicities might be avoided by reducing the maintenance infusion prior to the achievement of steady state.

Prediction of Plasma Levels Following Discontinuation of an Infusion. See Fig. 23. The plasma concentration any time after an infusion is discontinued (t_2) can be estimated by multiplying the measured or predicted plasma concentration at the time the infusion is discontinued by the fraction of drug remaining at t_2.

$$\begin{array}{l}\textbf{Fraction of Drug}\\ \textbf{Remaining at } t_2\end{array} = (e^{-Kdt_2}) \qquad \textbf{(Eq. 34)}$$

Plasma Conc. at t_2 = (Plasma Conc. at t_1)(Fract. Remaining at t_2)

$$= \frac{\textbf{(S)(F)(Dose/}\tau\textbf{)}}{\textbf{Cl}} \times (1 - e^{-Kdt_1})(e^{-Kdt_2}) \qquad \textbf{(Eq. 35)}$$

While Eq. 35 looks complicated, it is only a variation of the first-order equation which describes elimination:

$$\text{Cp} = (\text{Cp}^0)(e^{-Kdt}) \qquad \text{(Eq. 22)}$$

where Cp^0 is the concentration at the beginning of the interval which in this case is the point at which the infusion was discontinued. See Fig. 23.

To illustrate, the expected theophylline concentration 8 hours after discontinuing an aminophylline infusion of 100 mg/hour that had been administered for 16 hours to a patient with a theophylline clearance of 2.8 L/hour and a half-life of 8 hours (Kd of 0.087 hr^{-1}) would be 10.7 mg/L. The calculations could be done step by step as follows:

a) The expected steady state theophylline concentration resulting from an aminophylline infusion of 100 mg/hour to a patient with a theophylline clearance of 2.8 L/hr could be calculated using Eq. 31:

$$\text{Cpss ave} = \frac{(0.8)(1.0)(100 \text{ mg/hr})}{2.8 \text{ L/hr}}$$

$$= 28.6 \text{ mg/L}$$

b) The expected concentration after 16 hours of infusion (t_1) can be calculated using Eq. 32:

$$\text{Cp at } t_1 = (28.6 \text{ mg/L})(1 - e^{(-0.087 \text{ hrs}^{-1})(16 \text{ hrs})})$$

$$= (28.6 \text{ mg/L})(1 - e^{-1.392})$$

$$= (28.6 \text{ mg/L})(1 - 0.25)$$

$$= 21.45 \text{ mg/L}$$

c) The expected concentration 8 hours after the end of the infusion can be calculated using Eq. 35:

$$\text{Cp at } t_2 = (21.45 \text{ mg/L})(e^{(-0.087 \text{ hrs}^{-1})(8 \text{ hr})})$$

$$= (21.45 \text{ mg/L})(e^{-0.693})$$

$$= (21.45 \text{ mg/L})(0.5)$$

$$= 10.7 \text{ mg/L}$$

Dosing Interval (τ). The half-life can also be used to estimate the appropriate dosing interval (τ) for maintenance therapy. For example, if the goal of therapy is to minimize plasma fluctuations to no more than 50% between doses, the dosing interval

(τ) should be less than or equal to the half-life. The maintenance dose can be calculated using Eq. 15:

$$\text{Maintenance Dose} = \frac{(\text{Cl})(\text{Cpss ave})(\tau)}{(\text{S})(\text{F})} \qquad \text{(Eq. 15)}$$

If tau is less than or equal to the half-life of a drug, the calculated maintenance dose will produce plasma levels which will fluctuate by 50% or less during that dosing interval. The plasma levels will be above the average steady state plasma level for the first half of the dosing interval and below the average steady state plasma level during the second half of the dosing interval. See Fig. 19.

If the approximate half-life and dosing interval are known, one can determine the degree of change in plasma drug concentration which will occur over a dosing interval. Once the degree of fluctuation is known, one can then determine whether the primary determinant of plasma levels between dosing intervals is the volume of distribution or clearance. See following discussion.

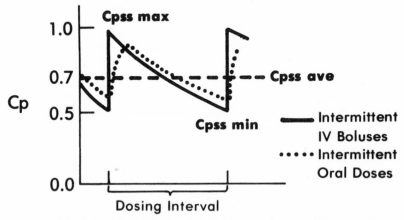

Fig. 19. **Plasma Level Time Curve for Intermittent Dosing at Steady State.** When the dosing interval is equal to the half-life, plasma concentrations are above the average steady state plasma concentration (Cpss ave) approximately 50% of the time and below Cpss ave approximately 50% of the time. Note that oral administration dampens the curve considerably and that the maximum concentration at steady state (Cpss max) occurs later and is lower than that produced by an IV bolus. The minimum concentration at steady state (Cpss min) is greater than that produced by IV bolus doses because of the effect of absorption.

In certain situations, the *dosing interval is much longer than the half-life,* and, for practical purposes, all of the drug is eliminated before the next dose. Therefore, each new dose is essentially a new loading dose. In this situation the peak concentration will be primarily determined by the volume of distribution because almost no drug is present from the previous dose.

Antibiotics are commonly dosed in this manner because the half-lives are so short that it is impractical to administer them every half-life. Additionally, the therapeutic index is usually so large that wide fluctuations in plasma level are acceptable. Furthermore, the therapeutic effect may require that the plasma level be above the minimal bactericidal or inhibitory concentration for only a brief period of time relative to the entire dosing interval.

When the *dosing interval is much shorter than the half-life,* the plasma level fluctuates very little over a dosing interval. When this is the case, the plasma level will be primarily determined by clearance. Digoxin and phenobarbital given orally and any drug administered by a constant infusion are good examples of such a situation. (Also see following section on Maximum and Minimum Concentrations.)

Determining the parameter which primarily affects plasma concentration for any given dosage regimen (when τ is longer or shorter than $t\frac{1}{2}$) is important because one then knows which parameters can be calculated reliably from the reported steady state plasma concentrations. For example, if a patient who had been taking a dose of 0.375 mg of digoxin daily had a reported steady state plasma concentration of 3.8 mg/L, one could reliably calculate the digoxin clearance for this patient using Eq. 14 because in this instance ($\tau \leqslant \leqslant t\frac{1}{2}$) clearance is the major determinant of the patient's plasma concentration. However, one could not reliably use the reported plasma concentration to calculate Vd and Kd as discussed later in the section on Maximum and Minimum Plasma Concentrations (See Eq. 39) because Vd is not the major determinant of plasma concentration when τ is much shorter than the half-life. One could then estimate a new maintenance dose for the patient described using the calculated clearance.

MAXIMUM AND MINIMUM PLASMA CONCENTRATIONS

In the clinical setting, it is often important to estimate the maximum (Cpss max or peak) and minimum (Cpss min or trough) plasma drug concentrations produced by a given dose of drug during the dosing interval at steady state. See Fig. 19. For example, while it is critical in gentamicin therapy to achieve a peak concentration which will inhibit bacterial growth, it is also important that the trough level be below a specified concentration to prevent dose-related toxicity.

For some drugs with a narrow therapeutic index (e.g., theophylline), it is useful to determine the degree of fluctuation in plasma drug concentration which will occur between doses. This can be particularly important if the dosing interval is longer than the half-life (i.e., fluctuations will be large) and Cpss min levels are being used to monitor therapy.

Most frequently, plasma specimens for drugs are drawn just prior to the next dose because Cpss min levels are the most reproducible. Although the plasma drug concentrations reported for these specimens are often treated as though they are average steady state levels (Cpss ave), more accurate estimates of a patient's pharmacokinetic parameters for the drug in question can be obtained using Eq. 39 which describes Cpss min.

The **maximum plasma drug concentration** can be calculated from Eq. 36 if the dose, bioavailability (F), volume of distribution (Vd), and elimination rate constant (Kd) are known:

$$\text{Cpss max} = \frac{\Delta \text{Cpss}}{\substack{\text{Fraction of Drug} \\ \text{Lost in } \tau}} \qquad \text{(Eq. 36)}$$

$$= \frac{\dfrac{(S)(F)(\text{Dose})}{Vd}}{(1 - e^{-Kd\tau})}$$

Where Δ Cpss and (S)(F)(Dose)/Vd represent the change in drug concentration which occurs over the dosing interval and $(1 - e^{-Kd\tau})$ represents the fraction of drug which is lost in the dosing interval. This equation assumes that the drug's absorption and distribution rates are rapid in relation to the dosing interval. This assumption is satisfactory for most drugs; however, digoxin and procainamide are notable exceptions.[1]

The **minimum plasma drug concentration** can be determined by subtracting Δ Cpss or the magnitude of change in plasma concentration in one dosing interval from the maximum plasma concentration:

$$\textbf{Cpss min} = \textbf{Cpss max} - \Delta \textbf{ Cpss}$$

$$= \textbf{Cpss max} - \frac{\textbf{(S)(F)(Dose)}}{\textbf{Vd}} \qquad \text{(Eq. 37)}$$

Alternatively, Cpss min can be calculated by multiplying Cpss max by the fraction of drug which remains at the end of the dosing interval $(e^{-Kd\tau})$:

$$\textbf{Cpss min} = \textbf{(Cpss max)}(e^{-Kd\tau}) \qquad \text{(Eq. 38)}$$

Substituting Eq. 36 for Cpss max into Eq. 38 enables one to calculate Cpss min if only the dose, elimination rate constant (Kd), half-life, and bioavailability (F) are known:

$$\textbf{Cpss min} = \frac{\dfrac{\textbf{(S)(F)(Dose)}}{\textbf{Vd}}}{(1 - e^{-Kd\tau})} \times (e^{-Kd\tau}) \qquad \text{(Eq. 39)}$$

One note of caution: When the absorption rate or a short dosing interval relative to the half-life significantly dampen the plasma drug concentration versus time curve (as for procainamide or digoxin), it may be more reasonable to assume that Cpss min is a close approximation of the average steady state concentration (Cpss ave) and to use Eq. 14 to calculate the

---

1. For *digoxin,* the observed peak concentration will be greater than predicted by the calculation for Cpss max because drug distribution into tissue requires a minimum of 6 hours. For *procainamide,* the observed peak concentration will be lower than that predicted on the basis of a calculated Cpss max because absorption is slow relative to the dosing interval and half-life for the drug. This tends to blunt or dampen the peak and trough levels of procainamide because elimination begins before all of the drug enters the body. For most drugs, the time required to reach peak concentrations after oral administration is between one and two hours.

patient's pharmacokinetic parameters. See Fig. 19. The Kd and Vd values which can be calculated from the Cpss min equation may be misleading in this instance, because when the dosing interval is much shorter than the half-life or when there is a substantial blunting of the plasma drug concentration versus time curve, plasma levels are primarily determined by clearance. Although the product of the Vd and Kd terms obtained by this method may closely approximate clearance, there can be no confidence in the Vd and Kd values per se because Vd and therefore Kd may vary independently of the clearance. Also see the section on Elimination Rate Constant and Half-life.

INTERPRETATION OF PLASMA DRUG CONCENTRATIONS

Plasma drug concentrations are measured in the clinical setting to determine whether a therapeutic or toxic concentration has been produced by a given dosage regimen. This is based upon the premise that the plasma drug concentrations reflect drug concentrations at the receptor and can therefore be correlated with pharmacologic response. This is not always the case and several factors must be evaluated before this assumption can be made. Some of the confounding situations which occur commonly in the clinical setting are discussed below.

Time of Plasma Sampling

Before any plasma drug concentration is interpreted, it is essential to know when the sample was obtained in relation to the last dose administered and the initiation of the drug regimen. As discussed earlier, if a plasma sample is obtained before distribution of the drug into tissue is complete (e.g., digoxin), the plasma concentration will be higher than predicted on the basis of dose and response. Peak (Cpss max) plasma levels are used by some clinicians to aid in the evaluation of the dose of antibiotics used to treat severe life-threatening infections. Although peak concentrations for many drugs occur one to two hours after the dose is administered, factors such as slow or delayed absorption can significantly delay the peak time. Clearly, a large error in the estimation of Cpss max can occur

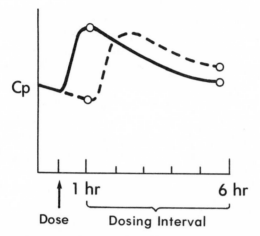

Fig. 20. Schematic Representation of the Effect of Delayed Absorption (- - - - -) on Plasma Level Measurements. Note the magnitude of error at one hour (theoretical time to reach Cpss max) as compared to six hours (Cpss min).

if the plasma sample is obtained at the wrong time (see Fig. 20). For these reasons, routine drug plasma levels should be drawn just prior to the next dose. These levels are more valid because they are less likely to be influenced by absorption and distribution problems.

To assess the full therapeutic response of a given dosage regimen, plasma levels should not be obtained until steady state is achieved. Commonly, drug doses are increased or decreased on the basis of drug concentrations measured from plasma samples obtained while the drug is still accumulating. The potentially disastrous consequences of these adjustments are obvious. Nevertheless in some clinical situations it *is* valid to measure drug levels prior to steady state. For example, pharmacokinetic parameters for a drug administered to a severely ill patient may change so rapidly that extrapolations made from a reported plasma concentration may not be valid from one day to the next. Similarly, if there is reason to suspect that the pharmacokinetic parameters in a given patient are likely to differ from those reported in the literature (e.g., lidocaine in a patient with congestive heart failure) it is valid to obtain plasma samples prior to steady state to assure that toxic or subtherapeutic levels will not result from the current dose. If possible, plasma samples should be drawn after two half-lives have passed, because a clearance value calculated from drug levels obtained less than one half-life after a dose has been initiated is very sensitive to small differences in the volume of distribution and minor assay errors.

Assay Specificity

The accuracy and specificity of the assay used by the laboratory measuring the plasma drug concentrations is critical to the establishment of a therapeutic range. Many drug assays measure both the unchanged, active drug and inactive metabolites. For example, the non-specific protein precipitate assay for quinidine which was used in many earlier studies measures quinidine as well as a number of relatively inactive metabolites and has a therapeutic range of 4 to 8 mcg/ml. This is in contrast to the relatively low therapeutic ranges reported for the more specific double extraction (26,35) and high performance liquid chromatography (HPLC) (10,181) assays for quinidine (2 to 5 mcg/ml and 1 to 4 mcg/ml respectively). It should be emphasized that because measured plasma drug concentrations which are obtained from more specific assays result in *lower* values, the Vd and clearance values derived from these concentrations are *higher* than those derived from less specific assay measurements (See Eq. 9 and 13). Pharmacokinetic parameters which have been derived from assays with differing specificities are not interchangeable.

For assays which measure the parent compound only, it is important to determine the pharmacologic activity and pharmacokinetic behavior of the metabolites. Many drugs have *active metabolites* which may affect a patient's pharmacologic response (See Table 4); this would not be predicted by an assay that measures only the parent compound. Procainamide has an active metabolite, N-acetylprocainamide (NAPA), which accumulates to rather high concentrations in patients with renal failure (29). In this case, an assay that measures only procainamide would underestimate the pharmacologic response of the patient.

Table 4
EXAMPLES OF DRUGS WITH ACTIVE METABOLITES

Amitriptyline
Carbamazepine
Chlordiazepoxide
Chlorpromazine
Chlorpropamide
Diazepam
Lidocaine
Procainamide
Propranolol
Warfarin

Adapted from reference 11.

Assay Error and Patient Factors

It cannot be overemphasized that, at best, drug levels are only an indirect indication of therapeutic response. Whenever possible, one should evaluate the patient's clinical response directly. If drug levels and clinical response do not correlate as predicted, it may be due to an error in the reported value. Similarly, factors unique to the patient such as concurrent disease states or antagonistic drug therapy may alter one's interpretation of the plasma drug concentration. For example, it is a common clinical observation that higher than usual plasma concentrations of digoxin are required to achieve a clinical response in patients with atrial fibrillation and in patients receiving propranolol. Furthermore, when plasma protein binding is decreased, therapeutic responses can be achieved with lower than usual therapeutic concentrations. The formation of aberrant metabolites and tachyphylaxis are other reasons for a lack of correlation between plasma drug concentration and therapeutic response.

SELECTING THE APPROPRIATE EQUATION

It is often difficult for the neophyte clinical pharmacokineticist to determine which of the many equations should be used to solve specific clinical problems. A technique which is used by this author to avoid the use of inappropriate equations is to draw a graphical representation of the plasma drug concentration versus time curve which would be expected on the basis of the dosage regimen the patient is receiving. Once the graph is drawn and the plasma concentration is visualized, mathematical equations which describe the drug's pharmacokinetic behavior are selected. To facilitate this process a series of typical plasma level time curves and their corresponding formulas are presented in Figures 21 through 25.

In the case where a **loading dose or a bolus of drug** has been administered (See Fig. 21), it is possible to determine the initial plasma concentration (Cp^0) by rearranging the "loading dose" equation (Eq. 10):

$$Cp^0 = \frac{(S)(F)(\text{Loading Dose})}{Vd} \qquad \text{(Eq. 40)}$$

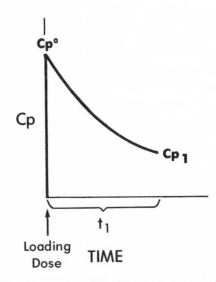

Fig. 21. Graphical Representation of the Change in Plasma Level Which Occurs Over Time Following a Loading Dose. Cp^0 represents the initial concentration and Cp_1 represents the concentration any interval of time (t_1) after the dose has been administered. Assume a one compartment model and rapid absorption if the drug is given orally.

$$Cp^0 = \frac{(S)(F)(\text{Loading Dose})}{Vd} \qquad \text{(Eq. 40)}$$

$$Cp_1 = \frac{(S)(F)(\text{Loading Dose})}{Vd} \times (e^{-Kdt_1}) \qquad \text{(Eq. 41)}$$

One can also determine a subsequent plasma level (Cp_1) any time (t_1) after the dose has been administered using a variation of the equation which describes first-order elimination (Eq. 22):

$$Cp_1 = (Cp^0)(e^{-Kdt_1})$$

$$= \frac{(S)(F)(Loading\ Dose)}{Vd} \times (e^{-Kdt_1}) \qquad (Eq.\ 41)$$

The plasma concentration versus time curve produced by a **continuous infusion which has been administered until steady state has been achieved** is represented by Fig. 22.

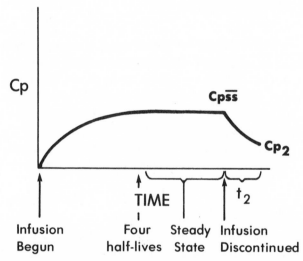

Fig. 22. **Graphical Representation of the Plasma Concentration Versus Time Curve Which Results When an Infusion is Continued until Steady State is Reached and Then Discontinued.** Cpss ave ($\overline{Cpss}$) is the steady state concentration and Cp_2 is the concentration at any interval of time (t_2) after the infusion has been discontinued.

$$Cpss\ ave = \frac{(S)(F)(Dose/\tau)}{Cl} \qquad (Eq.\ 31)$$

$$Cp_2 = \frac{(S)(F)(Dose/\tau)}{Cl} \times (e^{-Kdt_2}) \qquad (Eq.\ 42)$$

The curve which represents a change in the plasma concentration after the infusion has been discontinued is also represented in Fig. 21. The average steady state concentration (Cpss ave) which will be produced by the infusion, as well as the concentration (Cp_2) produced any time (t_2) after the infusion has been discontinued can be calculated using Eq. 31 and a variation of the first-order elimination equation (Eq. 22). (Also see discussion of Eq. 30–35):

$$\text{Cpss ave} = \frac{(S)(F)(Dose/\tau)}{Cl} \qquad \text{(Eq. 31)}$$

$$Cp_2 = (\text{Cpss ave})(e^{-Kdt_2}) \quad \text{or}$$

$$Cp_2 = \frac{(S)(F)(Dose/\tau)}{Cl} \times (e^{-Kdt_2}) \qquad \text{(Eq. 42)}$$

When an **infusion is initiated and discontinued *before* steady state is achieved** (less than four half-lives) the plasma level time curve can be described as depicted in Fig. 23. When this situation occurs it is possible to approximate the concentration (Cp_1) which is achieved by the infusion at any time (t_1) after the infusion was begun and the concentration (Cp_2) which results any time (t_2) after the infusion was discontinued by using Eq. 32 and 35. Also refer to earlier discussion of Eq. 30–35.

When a patient is given a **loading dose followed by an infusion** the plasma concentration (Cp_1) at any time (t_1) can be calculated by summing the equations which describe the loading dose at t_1 and the infusion at t_1. Refer to Fig. 21 and Fig. 23 up to Cp_1.

$$Cp_1 = \left[\frac{(S)(F)(\text{Loading Dose})}{Vd} \times (e^{-Kdt_1}) \right] + \left[\frac{(S)(F)(Dose/\tau)}{Cl} \times (1 - e^{-Kdt_1}) \right]$$

Note that Dose/τ in the second portion of the above equation represents the infusion rate. It is important to recall in this situation that the loading dose is eliminated according to first order kinetics just as described in Fig. 21 even when a maintenance infusion is initiated. This must be taken into account when predicting a plasma concentration. In other words, the maintenance infusion is accumulating while the concentration resulting from the loading dose is diminishing. See Fig. 24.

When a drug is administered **intermittently at regular dosing intervals until steady state** is achieved (at least four half-lives) the average concentration, the maximum concentration and the minimum concentration between dosing intervals can be approximated using Equations 31, 36, and 39. Fig. 25 depicts the plasma concentration versus time curve which occurs with this type of dosing regimen. Also see section on Maximum and Minimum Plasma Concentrations.

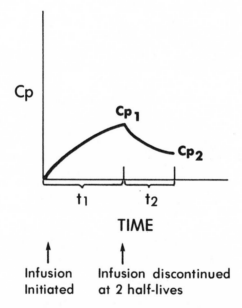

Fig. 23. Graphical Representation of an Infusion Which is Discontinued *Prior To* Steady State. Cp_1 is a concentration which is achieved any time (t_1) after the infusion is initiated and Cp_2 is a concentration which results any interval of time (t_2) after the infusion has been discontinued.

$$Cp_1 = \frac{(S)(F)(Dose/\tau)}{Cl} \times (1 - e^{-Kdt_1}) \qquad \text{(Eq. 32)}$$

$$Cp_2 = \frac{(S)(F)(Dose/\tau)}{Cl} \times (1 - e^{-Kdt_1}) \times (e^{-Kdt_2}) \qquad \text{(Eq. 35)}$$

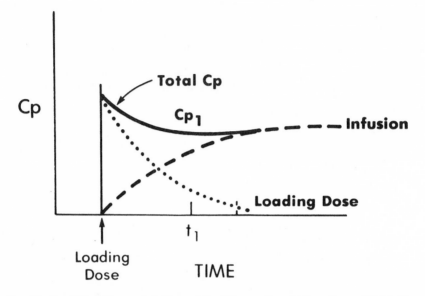

Fig. 24. Graphical Representation of the Plasma Level Time Curve Which Results from a Loading Dose Followed by a Maintenance Infusion. Note that the curve represents a summation of a loading dose curve ($\cdots$) and an infusion curve ($----$). Cp_1 is the concentration any time (t_1) after the loading dose has been administered and after the maintenance infusion has been initiated.

$$Cp_1 = \left[\frac{(S)(F)(\text{Loading Dose})}{Vd} \times (e^{-Kdt_1}) \right] + \left[\frac{(S)(F)(\text{Dose}/\tau)}{Cl} \times (1 - e^{-Kdt_1}) \right]$$

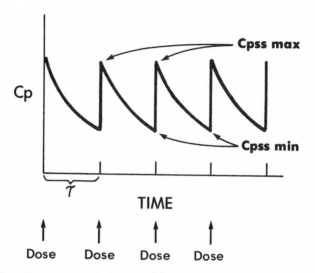

Fig. 25. Graphical Representation of the Steady State Plasma Concentration Versus Time Curve Which Occurs When Drugs are Given Intermittently at Regular Dosing Intervals. Note that any maximum concentration (Cpss max) is interchangeable with another maximum and any minimum concentration (Cpss min) is interchangeable with another minimum.

$$\text{Cpss ave} = \frac{(S)(F)(\text{Dose}/\tau)}{Cl} \qquad \text{(Eq. 31)}$$

$$\text{Cpss max} = \frac{(S)(F)(\text{Dose})/Vd}{(1-e^{-Kd\tau})} \qquad \text{(Eq. 36)}$$

$$\text{Cpss min} = \frac{(S)(F)(\text{Dose})/Vd}{(1-e^{-Kd\tau})} \times (e^{-Kd\tau}) \qquad \text{(Eq. 39)}$$

CREATININE CLEARANCE (Cl_{Cr})

Since many drugs are partially or totally eliminated by the kidney, an accurate estimation of creatinine clearance is crucial to the application of pharmacokinetics to drug therapy. The creatinine clearance is considered by most clinicians to be the most accurate test of renal function. In the actual clinical setting, however, an accurate Cl_{Cr} is difficult to obtain because it is based upon a 24-hour collection of urine. Frequently, the urine collection is inaccurate because a portion is accidentally discarded, or the time of collection is shorter or longer than requested. An incomplete collection will result in a gross underestimation of renal function (34). Furthermore, the method is expensive and time-consuming. Because decisions with regard to drug dosing must often be made quickly, several authors have suggested a variety of methods by which Cl_{Cr} can be estimated using a serum creatinine value.

Before discussing these, the basic pharmacokinetics of creatinine will be reviewed. This topic is presented in far more detail elsewhere (14,34). Creatinine is a metabolic by-product of muscle and its rate of formation (R_A) is primarily determined by an individual's muscle mass or lean body weight. It varies, therefore, with age (lower in the elderly) and sex (lower in the females) (30,32,47). For any given individual, the rate of creatinine production is constant. Once it is released from muscle into plasma, creatinine is excreted almost exclusively by the kidney through glomerular filtration. Any decrease in the glomerular filtration rate ultimately results in a rise in the serum creatinine level until a new steady state is reached and the *amount* of creatinine cleared per day equals the rate of production. In other words, at steady state, the rate in must equal the rate out. Since the rate of creatinine production *remains constant,* as renal clearance diminishes, the serum creatinine must rise until the product of the clearance and the serum creatinine again equals the rate of production. This concept is represented by Eq. 13 which was discussed earlier in the section on Clearance:

$$R_A = (Cl)(Cpss\ ave) \qquad \text{(Eq. 13)}$$

where R_A is the rate of creatinine production, Cl is creatinine clearance, and Cpss ave is a steady state serum creatinine level or $SrCr_{ss}$.

The degree to which a *steady state* serum creatinine rises is *inversely* proportional to the fall in creatinine clearance, so that a new creatinine clearance can be estimated by multiplying a normal Cl_{Cr} value by the fraction increase in the serum creatinine: Normal $SrCr/SrCr_{ss}$. For the 70 kg man, it can be assumed that the normal SrCr is 1.0 mg/dl and that the corresponding Cl_{Cr} is 100 ml/min:

$$\text{New Cl}_{Cr} = (100 \text{ ml/min}) \left(\frac{1.0 \text{ mg/dl}}{SrCr_{ss}} \right) \qquad \text{(Eq. 43)}$$

On the basis of this concept, one can see that each time the serum creatinine doubles, the creatinine clearance falls by one-half and that small changes in the serum creatinine at low levels are of much greater consequence than large changes in the serum creatinine at high levels. To illustrate, if a patient whose normal serum creatinine is 1.0 mg/dl is reported to have a new steady state serum creatinine of 2.0 mg/dl, the creatinine clearance has dropped from 100 ml/min to 50 ml/min. However, if a patient with chronic renal failure had a usual serum creatinine of 8.0 mg/dl (Cl_{Cr} = 12.5 ml/min), an increase in the serum creatinine to 16 mg/dl would result in a drop in the Cl_{Cr} by 6.25 ml/min.

This approach to the estimation of Cl_{Cr} from $SrCr_{ss}$ is reasonably satisfactory as long as the patient's daily creatinine production is average (i.e., 20 mg/kg/day), the serum creatinine is at steady state (i.e., not rising or falling), and the patient weighs approximately 70 kg.

To account for any changes in creatinine production and clearance which may result from a difference in body size, Eq. 43 can be modified to compensate for any deviation in body surface area (BSA) from the 70 kg man (1.73 m^2):

$$\text{New Cl}_{Cr} = (100 \text{ ml/min}) \left(\frac{1.0 \text{ mg/dl}}{SrCr_{ss}} \right) \left(\frac{\text{Patient's BSA}}{1.73 m^2} \right) \quad \text{(Eq. 44)}$$

Table 5
EXPECTED DAILY CREATININE PRODUCTION FOR MALES

Age (Years)	Daily Creatinine Production (mg/kg/day)
20–29	24
30–39	22
40–49	20
50–59	19
60–69	17
70–79	14
80–89	12
90–99	9

Adapted from reference 47.

The patient's BSA can be obtained from a nomogram (See Appendix I) or estimated from Eq. 16.

A disadvantage of this method is that many elderly or female patients do not have a "normal" creatinine of 1.0 mg/dl. Therefore, it may be erroneous to assume in these individuals that a SrCr of 1.0 mg/dl is indicative of normal renal function.

As patients become older, their muscle mass represents a smaller proportion of their total weight and creatinine production is decreased. See Table 5. The following method for estimating Cl_{Cr} from $SrCr_{ss}$ compensates for decreased creatinine production with age and sex (32):

$$Cl_{Cr} \text{ for males (ml/min/70 kg)} = \frac{98 - 0.8(\text{age} - 20)}{SrCr} \qquad \text{(Eq. 45)}$$

$$Cl_{Cr} \text{ for females (ml/min/70 kg)} = 0.9 \left[\frac{98 - 0.8(\text{age} - 20)}{SrCr} \right] \text{(Eq. 46)}$$

Estimating Time to Reach a Steady State Serum Creatinine Level

All of the above methods for estimating Cl_{Cr} require that the serum creatinine be at steady state. When patients have a sudden change in renal function, some period of time will be required to achieve a new steady state serum creatinine. It is important to estimate how long it will take for SrCr to reach steady state because if a rising serum creatinine is used in any of the previous equations, the patient's creatinine clearance will be overestimated.

As presented earlier, half-life is a function of both the volume of distribution and clearance. If the Vd for creatinine (42 L) is assumed to remain constant, the time required to reach 95% of steady state in patients with 50, 25, and 10% of normal renal functions has been estimated to be 1.07, 2.15 and 6.7 days respectively (24). Because it is difficult to estimate the percentage loss in renal function clinically, it has been suggested that two serum creatinines be obtained at 12 hour intervals. If there is an increase in the serum creatinine by 0.2 mg/dl or more, then it is likely that steady state has not been achieved. The likelihood that one is dealing with a non-steady state level increases as the absolute renal function diminishes because it takes longer for the serum creatinine to reach steady state.

Evaluating Creatinine Clearance Values

The accuracy of the reported creatinine clearance is highly dependent upon the adequacy of the urine collection. Therefore the completeness of the urine collection should always be checked by comparing the expected creatinine excretion with the amount actually collected. At steady state, rate in (creatinine production) equals rate out (creatinine excretion). If the amount collected differs significantly from the predicted production, the reported creatinine clearance is likely to be inaccurate. The patient's age, sex, and muscle mass should be considered in estimating the expected production of creatinine, since increasing age and smaller muscle mass will reduce the expected production rate. See Table 5.

This principle will be illustrated using the following example: The data below were reported for a 50 kg patient for whom a Cl_{Cr} was ordered.

Total collection time: 24 hours
Urine volume: 1200 ml
Urine creatinine concentration: 42 mg/dl
Serum creatinine: 1.5 mg/dl
Creatinine clearance: 23 ml/min (Uncorrected)
          30 ml/min (Corrected)

To determine whether the collection was complete, the total amount of creatinine collected in the 24-hour period should first be calculated:

Amount of
Creatinine = (Urine Vol./24 hrs)(Urine Creatinine Conc.) (Eq. 47)
Excreted

$$= (1200 \ ml/24 \ hrs)(42 \ mg/100 \ ml)$$

$$= 504 \ mg \ creatinine/24 \ hrs$$

Since the patient weighs 50 kg, the apparent creatinine production per day can be calculated by dividing the total amount of creatinine excreted by his weight:

Apparent Rate of
Creatinine Production $= \dfrac{\text{Amount of Creatinine Excreted}}{\text{Patient's Weight}}$ (Eq. 48)
per Day

$$= \frac{504 \ mg \ creatinine/24 \ hrs}{50 \ kg}$$

$$= 10.08 \ mg/kg/day$$

This apparent production rate of creatinine of approximately 10 mg/kg/day is considerably less than the normal production rate of 20 mg/kg/day. Therefore, the collection was probably incomplete, resulting in a reported value for creatinine clearance which was much less than the patient's actual Cl_{Cr}. On the other hand, if the patient has a very small muscle mass because he is poorly developed, atrophied, or elderly, the collection may be considered adequate and the reported creatinine clearance of 23 ml/min accurate.

As depicted in the patient's data above, both uncorrected and corrected creatinine clearance values are frequently reported by clinical laboratories. The "uncorrected" value usually represents the patient's actual creatinine clearance and the "corrected" value is what the patient's creatinine clearance would be if he or she were 70 kg or 1.73 m^2.

ALGORITHM FOR EVALUATING AND INTERPRETING PLASMA LEVELS

STEP 1. INITIAL DATA COLLECTION

Before one can interpret the patient's pharmacokinetic parameters or plasma drug levels, appropriate information must be collected so that factors which may influence drug absorption and disposition can be considered.

Relevant Physical Data, Medical and Surgical History: Height, weight, age, sex, race, current diseases and symptoms.

Relevant Laboratory Data

Renal Function: SrCr, BUN, Cl_{Cr} (Is the collection complete?)

Hepatic Function: Serum albumin, bilirubin, prothrombin time, serum enzymes.

Protein Binding: Plasma protein concentration. Acidic drugs—Albumin. Basic drugs—? Globulins. Evaluate displacing factors such as drugs or presence of uremia.

Thyroid function

Drug Administration History

Collect dosing data (dose, frequency, and route) for 3–5 half-lives. Consider history prior to admission as well as during hospital stay.

It is critical to determine the **exact** time of administration for those doses taken just prior to drug level sampling.

Time of Sampling Relative to the Last Dose

The best time to sample is usually just prior to the next dose. For drugs with a short half-life, peak and trough levels may be appropriate. Avoid absorption and distribution phase when peak levels are obtained.

(continue on next page)

63

STEP 2. EVALUATION OF REPORTED PLASMA LEVELS

Non-Steady State Plasma Concentration

The plasma level must be evaluated by considering the contribution of each dose at the time the plasma sample was obtained. Use Eq. 41 for each bolus dose. If several different infusion rates have been used during the accumulation period, Equations 32 or 35 should be used for each infusion rate.

Cp is greater than expected:

See List A

Vd may be less than expected.

Sample was obtained during distribution phase.

Cp is less than expected:

See List B

Vd may be greater than expected.

The sample was obtained too soon after the dose was administered and absorption was not yet complete.

List A

When drug concentrations are greater than expected, consider:

1. Increased bioavailability. This is only important if the drug's bioavailability is usually low.

2. Noncompliance. Intake is greater than prescribed.

3. Decreased clearance.

4. Increased plasma protein binding. Changes in plasma protein binding will be most important if α is ≤ 0.1. It is unlikely to be significant if α is >0.5. Increased plasma protein binding will also decrease the volume of distribution and clearance of most drugs.

List B

When drug concentrations are less than expected, consider:

1. Decreased bioavailability.

2. Noncompliance. Intake is less than prescribed.

3. Increased clearance.

4. Decreased plasma protein binding. Changes in plasma protein binding will be most important if α is ≤ 0.1 and are unlikely to be significant if α is >0.5. Decreased plasma binding will also increase the volume of distribution and the clearance of most drugs.

64

Has the patient been receiving
constant dosing for more than 3
to 4 half-lives prior to obtaining
the plasma sample?

NO

YES

**Drug Concentration
Represents A Steady State
Level.**

Is the drug being administered as
a constant infusion, as a delayed
release product, or is the dosing
interval much less than the drug
half-life?

NO

See Page 66

YES

Drug concentration can be evaluated as
Cpss ave. Eq. 31.

Cpss ave is greater than expected:

See List A

Sample may have been
collected during the
distribution phase.

Cpss ave is less than expected:

See List B

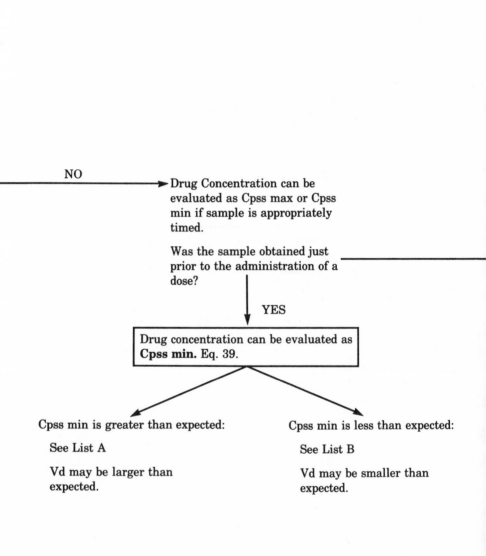

NO → Drug Concentration can be evaluated as Cpss max or Cpss min if sample is appropriately timed.

Was the sample obtained just prior to the administration of a dose?

YES

Drug concentration can be evaluated as **Cpss min.** Eq. 39.

Cpss min is greater than expected:

  See List A

  Vd may be larger than expected.

Cpss min is less than expected:

  See List B

  Vd may be smaller than expected.

List A	List B
When drug concentrations are greater than expected, consider:	When drug concentrations are less than expected, consider:
1. Increased bioavailability. This is only important if the drug's bioavailability is usually low.	1. Decreased bioavailability.
	2. Noncompliance. Intake is less than prescribed.
2. Noncompliance. Intake is greater than prescribed.	3. Increased clearance.
3. Decreased clearance.	4. Decreased plasma protein binding. Changes in plasma protein binding will be most important if α is ≤ 0.1 and are unlikely to be significant if α is > 0.5. Decreased plasma binding will also increase the volume of distribution and the clearance of most drugs.
4. Increased plasma protein binding. Changes in plasma protein binding will be most important if α is ≤ 0.1. It is unlikely to be significant if α is > 0.5. Increased plasma protein binding will also decrease the volume of distribution and clearance of most drugs.	

NO

If sample was obtained one to two hours after an oral dose or upon completion of a short intravenous infusion, concentration may be evaluated as **Cpss max.** Eq. 36.

Cpss max is greater than expected:

See List A

Sample may have been obtained during the distribution phase.

Vd may be smaller than expected.

Cpss max is less than expected:

See List B

Vd may be larger than expected.

Absorption of last dose was delayed or slower than expected.

67

PART TWO

2

Digoxin

Digoxin is an inotropic agent which is primarily used in the treatment of congestive heart failure and atrial fibrillation. It is incompletely absorbed and a substantial fraction is cleared by the kidneys. Because it has a relatively long elimination half-life, an oral loading dose of approximately 1.0–1.5 mg/70 kg is administered prior to a usual maintenance dose of 0.25 mg. It is generally prescribed orally as tablets and is given once daily. Dosage adjustments are critical in any patient who is being converted from parenteral to oral therapy or vice versa; a patient who has concurrent renal impairment, congestive heart failure, or thyroid abnormalities; or a patient who is also taking quinidine.

Therapeutic Plasma Concentrations

While there is considerable variation between patients, plasma digoxin concentrations of approximately 1 to 2 ng/ml (mcg/L) are considered to be within the therapeutic range (54,55). There is evidence that using pharmacokinetics to adjust the dosing regimen can reduce the incidence of toxicity (36,45,55,56).

Bioavailability

The bioavailability (F) of digoxin tablets ranges from 0.5 to 0.9. Many clinicians use a bioavailability of 0.7 or 0.8 to minimize any possibility of overdosing the patient. The bioavailability of 0.62 used in this text was selected as an estimate of the average bioavailability figures reported in the literature (31).

Volume of Distribution

The average volume of distribution (Vd) for digoxin is approximately 7.3 L/kg (42). This Vd is decreased in patients with renal

71

disease (Question 4), in hypothyroid patients (Question 12), and in patients who are taking quinidine (Question 14). It is increased in hyperthyroid patients (Question 12).

The way in which digoxin is distributed in the body must be considered in the interpretation of plasma levels. The distribution of digoxin follows a two compartment model (see Part One, section on Volume of Distribution: Two Compartment Model). This drug is distributed initially into the plasma compartment and then into a tissue compartment where it exerts its pharmacological effects on the myocardium. Since plasma samples are obtained from Vi, plasma digoxin levels do not accurately reflect the drug's pharmacologic effects until it is completely distributed into both compartments. Digoxin levels obtained prior to complete distribution are often misleading. Because the initial volume of distribution (Vi) is relatively small (approximately 1/10 Vt), high plasma levels are commonly reported immediately after a dose is administered; however, because the heart behaves as though it were in the second, or tissue compartment, these levels are not reflective of either therapeutic or toxic effects. In order to be meaningful, plasma levels should be obtained at least four hours after an intravenous dose (53) or six hours after an oral dose (51). Since the distribution half-life ($\alpha t^{1/2}$) is only about 35 minutes (66) the clinical effects of a dose may be observed much sooner. The myocardium experiences the effects of 75% of an intravenous dose after about one hour; however, a plasma sample taken at this time would be misleadingly high, because the remaining 25% of the dose which is not yet distributed would cause the drug concentration in the plasma to be quite high compared to what it would be after complete equilibrium is achieved between the two compartments. This is illustrated in Fig. 1.

KEY PARAMETERS	
Therapeutic Concentrations	1–2 ng/ml
F (Tablets)	0.62
F (Elixir)	0.8
Vd^a (at steady state)	7.3 L/kg
$Cl^{a,b}$	57 ml/min + 1.02 Cl_{Cr}
$\beta t^{1/2}$	2 days

[a] Altered by renal disease, thyroid disease, and quinidine. See text.
[b] Altered by congestive heart failure.

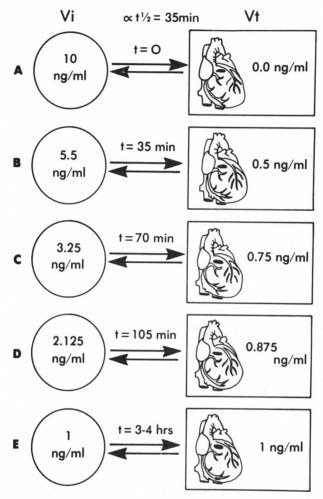

Fig. 1. A Theoretical Two Compartment Model for Digoxin. Note that the initial volume of distribution (Vi) is much smaller than the tissue volume of distribution (Vt). The myocardium or target organ behaves as though it were in Vt and therefore responds to the theoretical digoxin concentration in Vt. Following complete distribution, the concentration in Vi and Vt are assumed to be equal and the pharmacologic effect maximal. Fig. 1-A depicts digoxin distribution immediately following an intravenous bolus. All of the drug is in Vi and the plasma concentration is 10 ng/ml. Fig. 1-E depicts complete digoxin distribution. Note that the two compartments are in equilibrium and that the digoxin concentration in both Vi and Vt is 1 ng/ml. At this point, the plasma level accurately reflects the level in the tissue compartment. Figs. 1-B, 1-C and 1-D depict the relative digoxin concentrations in Vi and Vt after one, two and three distribution half-lives (αt½'s). Note that after three αt½'s that 87.5% of the pharmacologic effect is achieved; however, it is still much too early to obtain a digoxin level because the concentration in Vi is more than 100% higher than the final equilibrated concentration.

73

Clearance

Digoxin clearance varies considerably among individuals and should be estimated for each patient. Total digoxin clearance is the sum of its metabolic and renal clearance:

$$Cl_t = Cl_m + Cl_r \tag{Eq. 20}$$

In healthy individuals the metabolic clearance of digoxin is approximately 40 to 60 ml/min/70 kg, and the renal clearance is about equal to or a little less than the creatinine clearance. However, the presence of congestive heart failure reduces the metabolic clearance to about one-half its usual value and may slightly reduce the renal clearance of digoxin (6,57,58,65). (Also see Part One, section on Clearance).

Using the data from Shiener (6), the total digoxin clearance for a 70 kg (1.73 m²) patient can be calculated as follows:

without congestive heart failure (70 kg):

Total
Digoxin   (ml/min) = 57 ml/min + 1.02(Cl_{Cr})   (Eq. 49)
Clearance

with congestive heart failure (70 kg):

Total
Digoxin   (ml/min) = 23 ml/min + 0.88(Cl_{Cr})   (Eq. 50)
Clearance

Where Cl_{Cr} is the creatinine clearance in ml/min for a 70 kg patient. Creatinine clearance can be estimated from the patient's serum creatinine by use of Equation 45 or 46:

$$Cl_{Cr} \text{ for males (ml/min/70 kg)} = \frac{98 - 0.8(age - 20)}{SrCr} \tag{Eq. 45}$$

$$Cl_{Cr} \text{ for females (ml/min/70 kg)} = 0.9\left[\frac{98 - 0.8(age - 20)}{SrCr}\right] \tag{Eq. 46}$$

These and other methods for estimating digoxin clearance are illustrated in the questions which follow.

Elimination Half-life

The half-life for digoxin is approximately 2 days in patients with normal renal function. In anephric patients, the half-life increases to approximately 4 to 6 days. The increase in the half-life is less than might be expected because of the decreased volume of distribution associated with diminished renal function. See Question 4.

1. Estimate the digoxin loading dose that would be required to achieve a plasma concentration of 1.5 ng/ml (mcg/L) for an average 70 kg patient being treated for congestive heart failure.

Estimating a loading dose requires knowledge of the volume of distribution of the drug. In this case, the average Vd for digoxin, 7.3 L/kg, can be used (42). Using Eq. 10, the loading dose can be calculated as follows:

$$\text{Loading Dose} = \frac{(Vd)(Cp)}{(S)(F)} \qquad \text{(Eq. 10)}$$

$$= \frac{(7.3 \text{ L/kg})(70 \text{ kg})(1.5 \text{ mcg/L})}{(1)(0.62)}$$

$$= \frac{(511 \text{ L})(1.5 \text{ mcg/L})}{0.62}$$

$$= \frac{766.5 \text{ mcg}}{0.62}$$

$$= 1236.3 \text{ mcg}$$

or, approximately 1250 mcg.

In this case it was assumed that the loading dose was to be given orally as tablets. Therefore, the bioavailability (F) was assumed to be 0.62 (31). If the loading dose were to be given by the intravenous route, the bioavailability (F) would have been 1.0 and the calculated loading dose would have been 766.5 mcg (approximately 750 mcg). In both cases, S is 1.0 since digoxin is not administered as a salt.

2. How should this loading dose be divided, and what would be an appropriate interval between doses?

Loading doses of digoxin are almost always administered in divided doses so that the patient can be evaluated for toxicity and efficacy prior to receiving the total loading dose. If the patient appears to develop toxicity or is therapeutically controlled, the remainder of the calculated loading dose is withheld. The usual procedure is to give one-half of the calculated loading dose initially followed by one-fourth in six hours; the remaining fourth is administered six hours after the second dose.

Six hours is the usual interval between doses since it is the approximate time required for digoxin to be absorbed and distributed to the myocardium (51). Even following an intravenous injection, approximately two to four hours are required for a single dose of digoxin to exhibit its full effect (53). Also see Part One, section on Loading Dose.

3. Assuming the patient in Question 1 was a 50-year-old male who had a serum creatinine of 1.0 mg/dl, calculate a maintenance dose that would maintain the average plasma digoxin concentration at 1.5 ng/ml (mcg/L).

Since the objective is to achieve an average digoxin concentration at steady state (Cpss ave), it is appropriate to use Eq. 15 to calculate the maintenance dose:

$$\text{Maintenance Dose} = \frac{(\text{Cl})(\text{Cpss ave})(\tau)}{(\text{S})(\text{F})} \qquad \text{(Eq. 15)}$$

Assuming the dosing interval (τ) to be one day, the bioavailability (F) to be 0.62 for oral tablets and the fraction of the dose which is digoxin (S) to be 1.0, the clearance (Cl) is the only remaining factor to be calculated.

The *clearance* for this patient can be determined by use of Eq. 50:

$$\begin{array}{l}\text{Total} \\ \text{Digoxin} \\ \text{Clearance}\end{array} \text{(ml/min)} = 23\,\text{ml/min} + 0.88(\text{Cl}_{\text{Cr}}) \qquad \text{(Eq. 50)}$$

Although the *creatinine clearance* (Cl_{Cr}) for this patient is not known, it can easily be estimated from his serum creatinine by use of Eq. 45, assuming all the criteria for the use of this formula are met (e.g., serum creatinine is at steady state, patient's muscle mass is average for a 50-year-old male):

$$Cl_{Cr} \text{ for males (ml/min/70 kg)} = \frac{98 - 0.8(age - 20)}{SrCr} \quad \text{(Eq. 45)}$$

$$= \frac{98 - 0.8(50 - 20)}{1.0}$$

$$= \frac{98 - 24}{1.0}$$

$$= 74 \text{ ml/min}$$

This estimate of creatinine clearance can now be used to estimate the patient's total digoxin clearance:

$$\text{Total Digoxin Clearance (ml/min)} = 23 \text{ ml/min} + 0.88(Cl_{Cr}) \quad \text{(Eq. 50)}$$

$$= 23 \text{ ml/min} + 0.88(74 \text{ ml/min})$$

$$= 23 \text{ ml/min} + 65 \text{ ml/min}$$

$$= 88 \text{ ml/min}$$

This clearance could be used to calculate the maintenance dose in ng/min, but a maintenance dose stated in mcg/day is more practical. The clearance can be converted to L/day by multiplying by the number of minutes per day (1440 min/day) and dividing by the number of ml per liter (1000 ml/L):

$$Cl \text{ as L/day} = \frac{(Cl \text{ as ml/min})(1440 \text{ min/day})}{1000 \text{ ml/L}}$$

$$= \frac{(88 \text{ ml/min})(1440 \text{ min/day})}{1000 \text{ ml/L}}$$

$$= 126.7 \text{ L/day}$$

The maintenance dose can now be calculated using Eq. 15:

$$\text{Maintenance Dose} = \frac{(Cl)(Cpss\ ave)(\tau)}{(S)(F)} \qquad \text{(Eq. 15)}$$

$$= \frac{(126.7\ L/day)(1.5\ mcg/L)(1\ day)}{(1.0)(0.62)}$$

$$= \frac{190\ mcg/day}{0.62}$$

$$= 306.5\ mcg/day$$

$$= 0.3065\ mg/day$$

One could elect to give either 0.25 or 0.375 mg/day as these would be the most convenient dosage forms, or 0.25 and 0.375 mg could be alternated every other day for an average dose of 0.312 mg/day.

4. If the patient in Question 1 had a serum creatinine of 5 mg/dl would the estimated loading dose have been different?

For a number of years it was assumed that renal function influenced only the clearance of digoxin. Recent studies have indicated, however, that patients with decreased creatinine clearance also have a decreased volume of distribution for digoxin (6,33,42).

The relationship between volume of distribution, plasma concentration and amount of drug in the body is described by Eq. 9:

$$Vd = \frac{Ab}{Cp} \qquad \text{(Eq. 9)}$$

It is assumed that in patients with uremia digoxin in the tissue compartment is displaced, resulting in a smaller Vd and therefore a greater Cp:

$$\downarrow Vd = \frac{Ab}{\uparrow Cp} \qquad \text{(Eq. 9)}$$

There is some controversy as to the significance of this tissue displacement of digoxin. It has been shown that uremic patients have decreased myocardial concentrations relative to their plasma levels (59), and it has been suggested that because of the decreased myocardial concentration, uremic patients may actually require no change in loading dose (60). While there is no direct evidence as to whether or not it is appropriate to reduce the loading dose of digoxin in uremics, it is usually assumed that since increased plasma concentrations are associated with increased toxicities, the loading dose should be reduced.

Since very little digoxin is bound to plasma proteins (about 30%), a change in the desired plasma concentration due to displacement from plasma proteins is unlikely (61). (See Part One, section on Desired Plasma Concentration).

There are a number of ways to estimate the volume of distribution for digoxin in a patient with decreased renal function; Equations 51 and 52 are the most commonly used:

$$\text{Digoxin Volume of Distribution (L/70 kg)} = 226 + \frac{298(Cl_{Cr})}{29 + Cl_{Cr}} \tag{Eq. 51}$$

$$\text{Digoxin Volume of Distribution (L/70 kg)} = 269 + 3.12(Cl_{Cr}) \tag{Eq. 52}$$

Both of these equations are normalized to 70 kg and, therefore, require that the creatinine clearance (Cl_{Cr}) be expressed as ml/min/70 kg. If the patient is smaller or larger than 70 kg, the volume of distribution can be adjusted in proportion to the patient's body size. In addition, it is important to remember that the volumes of distribution for digoxin in uremic patients can vary considerably, so the values obtained from these equations should be considered as only rough estimates.

Using Eq. 45 the patient's creatinine clearance is determined to be approximately 15 ml/min:

$$Cl_{Cr} \text{ for males (ml/min/70 kg)} = \frac{98 - 0.8(age - 20)}{SrCr} \tag{Eq. 45}$$

$$= \frac{98 - 0.8(50 - 20)}{5.0}$$

$$= \begin{array}{l} 14.8 \text{ ml/min or} \\ \text{approximately 15 ml/min} \end{array}$$

Using this value in Eq. 51 and 52, the estimated volumes of distribution would be 327.6 L and 315.8 L respectively:

$$\text{Digoxin Volume of Distribution (L/70 kg)} = 226 + \frac{298(\text{Cl}_{\text{Cr}})}{29 + \text{Cl}_{\text{Cr}}} \qquad \text{(Eq. 51)}$$

$$= 226 + \frac{298(15)}{29 + 15}$$

$$= 226 + \frac{4470}{44}$$

$$= 327.6 \text{ L}$$

$$\text{Digoxin Volume of Distribution (L/70 kg)} = 269 + 3.12(\text{Cl}_{\text{Cr}}) \qquad \text{(Eq. 52)}$$

$$= 269 + 3.12(15)$$

$$= 269 + 46.8$$

$$= 315.8 \text{ L}$$

Since both of these approaches give similar estimates, either could be used. Eq. 52 appears to be useful over a wider range of creatinine clearance values, especially when the creatinine clearance is greater than 100 ml/min/70 kg (6,63).

If the volume of distribution is assumed to be 315.8 L (as calculated from Eq. 52), the estimated oral loading dose would be approximately 750 mcg:

$$\text{Loading Dose} = \frac{(\text{Vd})(\text{Cp})}{(\text{S})(\text{F})} \qquad \text{(Eq. 10)}$$

$$= \frac{(315 \text{ L})(1.5 \text{ mcg/L})}{(1.0)(0.62)}$$

$$= \frac{472 \text{ mcg}}{0.62}$$

$$= 762 \text{ mcg} \ (0.762 \text{ mg})$$

Again, as in Question 1, S and F are assumed to be 1.0 and 0.62 respectively. The total loading dose should be divided and administered as described in Question 2 to guard against the possibility that the volume of distribution is much smaller than anticipated or that the patient is more sensitive to the pharmacologic effects than expected. However, there is the possibility that the volume of distribution may be much larger than expected, and additional doses may have to be administered.

5. Estimate the daily dose that would maintain the average digoxin concentration at 1.5 ng/ml (mcg/L) in this same 50-year-old patient weighing 70 kg with a serum creatinine of 5.0 mg/dl.

As in Question 3, Eq. 15 would be used to estimate the maintenance dose:

$$\text{Maintenance Dose} = \frac{(\text{Cl})(\text{Cpss ave})(\tau)}{(\text{S})(\text{F})} \qquad \text{(Eq. 15)}$$

Using the creatinine clearance estimate of 15 ml/min from Question 4, the digoxin clearance can be estimated from Eq. 50 (for congestive heart failure):

$$\begin{aligned}
\text{Total Digoxin Clearance} &= 23 \text{ ml/min} + 0.88(\text{Cl}_{\text{Cr}}) \qquad \text{(Eq. 50)} \\
&= 23 \text{ ml/min} + 0.88(15 \text{ ml/min}) \\
&= 23 \text{ ml/min} + 13.2 \text{ ml/min} \\
&= 36.2 \text{ ml/min}
\end{aligned}$$

The digoxin clearance can be converted from ml/min to L/day as in Question 3:

$$\begin{aligned}
\text{Total Digoxin Clearance} &= \frac{(36.2 \text{ ml/min})(1440 \text{ min/day})}{1000 \text{ ml/L}} \\
&= 52.1 \text{ L/day}
\end{aligned}$$

Again, assuming S to be 1.0 and F to be 0.62 for digoxin tablets, the approximate daily dose would be 125 mcg/day (0.125 mg/day):

$$\text{Maintenance Dose} = \frac{(Cl)(\text{Cpss ave})(\tau)}{(S)(F)} \qquad \text{(Eq. 15)}$$

$$= \frac{(52 \text{ L/day})(1.5 \text{ mcg/L})(1 \text{ day})}{(1.0)(0.62)}$$

$$= \frac{78.2 \text{ mcg/day}}{0.62}$$

$$= \begin{array}{l}126 \text{ mcg/day or approximately} \\ 0.125 \text{ mg/day}\end{array}$$

6. Assume that the patient described above can take nothing by mouth and must be converted to daily intravenous doses of digoxin. Calculate an intravenous dose equivalent to the 0.125 mg tablets he ingests daily.

If the bioavailability of digoxin is assumed to be 0.62, the equivalent intravenous dose would be 0.0775 or 0.08 mg/day as calculated from Eq. 1 and 2:

$$\text{Amount of Drug Absorbed} = (F)(\text{Dose}) \qquad \text{(Eq. 1)}$$

$$= (0.62)(0.125 \text{ mg})$$

$$= 0.0775$$

$$\begin{array}{l}\text{Dose of New} \\ \text{Dosage Form}\end{array} = \frac{\begin{array}{c}\text{Amount of Drug Absorbed from} \\ \text{Current Dosage Form}\end{array}}{\text{F of New Dosage Form}} \qquad \text{(Eq. 2)}$$

$$= \frac{0.0775}{1}$$

$$= 0.0775 \text{ mg or } 0.08 \text{ mg}$$

If a dose reduction for the increased bioavailability of the intravenous dose were not made, substantially higher steady state digoxin concentrations would eventually be achieved (see Part One, Fig. 16).

7. A 62-year-old woman weighing 50 kg was admitted to the hospital for possible digoxin toxicity. Her serum creatinine was 3.0 mg/dl and her dosing regimen at home was 0.25 mg of digoxin each day for many months. The digoxin plasma concentration on admission was reported to be 4.0 ng/ml. How long will it take for the digoxin concentration to fall from 4.0 to 2.0 ng/ml?

The answer to this question requires a knowledge of the half-life (t½) or the elimination rate constant (Kd) which are dependent upon the clearance and volume of distribution of digoxin in this patient. The relationship between these parameters is described by Eq. 23 and 28:

$$Kd = \frac{Cl}{Vd} \qquad \text{(Eq. 23)}$$

$$t\frac{1}{2} = \frac{(0.693)(Vd)}{Cl} \qquad \text{(Eq. 28)}$$

Three basic steps are required to solve this problem: estimate clearance, estimate the Vd, and calculate the half-life.

Step 1. If we assume that the digoxin half-life is longer than the dosing interval, the observed digoxin plasma concentration should be reasonably representative of the average concentration at steady state (i.e., relatively independent of the volume of distribution; see Part One, section on Elimination Rate Constant and Half-Life). Therefore, the observed digoxin concentration could be used to estimate the patient's clearance:

$$Cl = \frac{(S)(F)(Dose/\tau)}{Cpss\ ave} \qquad \text{(Eq. 14)}$$

$$= \frac{(1.0)(0.62)(250\ mcg/day)}{4.0\ mcg/L}$$

$$= \frac{155\ mcg/day}{4.0\ mcg/L}$$

$$= 38.75\ L/day$$

This digoxin clearance of 38.75 L/day which was calculated from the patient's dosing history and observed plasma level is reasonably close to what would be expected for a 62-year-old woman weighing 50 kg and having a serum creatinine of 3.0 mg/dl. One could estimate digoxin clearance as in the previous questions by first determining the patient's creatinine clearance through use of Eq. 46 (for women):

$$Cl_{Cr} \text{ (ml/min)} = 0.9 \left[\frac{98 - 0.8(\text{age} - 20)}{SrCr} \right] \quad \text{(Eq. 46)}$$

$$= 0.9 \left[\frac{98 - 0.8(62 - 20)}{3.0} \right]$$

$$= 0.9 \left[\frac{98 - 33.6}{3.0} \right]$$

$$= 19.3 \text{ ml/min/70 kg}$$

and then using this estimation of Cl_{Cr} to determine the digoxin clearance by Eq. 50 (for congestive heart failure):

Total
Digoxin $= 23 \text{ ml/min} + 0.88(Cl_{Cr})$ (Eq. 50)
Clearance

$$= 23 \text{ ml/min} + 0.88(19.3 \text{ ml/min})$$

$$= 23 \text{ ml/min} + 17 \text{ ml/min}$$

$$= 40 \text{ ml/min/70 kg}$$

These values for Cl_{Cr} and digoxin clearance are based on the average 70 kg patient. The digoxin clearance for this patient should now be adjusted for her body size. Since she is relatively close to 70 kg, adjustments based on either weight or body surface area will give approximately the same results. If weight is used, the adjusted digoxin clearance would be:

$$40 \text{ ml/min} \left[\frac{50 \text{ kg}}{70 \text{ kg}} \right] = 28.6 \text{ ml/min}$$

Expressed as L/day:

$$\frac{(28.6 \text{ ml/min})(1440 \text{ min/day})}{1000 \text{ ml/L}} = 41 \text{ L/day}$$

This expected clearance of 41 L/day is reasonably close to the apparent clearance of 38.75 L/day which was obtained from the patient's dosing history and observed plasma level of 4.0 ng/ml. Had there been a substantial difference between the expected and apparent digoxin clearance, it would have been important to decide whether there was an error in the assumptions used in Eq. 14 (see Question 9) or whether the patient was really different from the average individual.

Step 2. The patient's digoxin volume of distribution can now be estimated using Eq. 52 and her estimated creatinine clearance (19.3 ml/min/70 kg):

$$\begin{array}{ll} \text{Digoxin} \\ \text{Volume of} & = 269 + 3.12(Cl_{Cr}) \\ \text{Distribution} \end{array} \qquad \text{(Eq. 52)}$$

$$= 269 + 3.12(19.3)$$

$$= 329.2 \text{ L}/70 \text{ kg}$$

Again, as in the clearance estimate, this equation is based upon a 70 kg patient and needs to be adjusted for her size. Therefore, the estimated digoxin volume of distribution is adjusted for her body weight of 50 kg:

$$329.2 \text{ L} \left[\frac{50 \text{ kg}}{70 \text{ kg}} \right] = 28.6 \text{ ml/min}$$

Step 3. The digoxin elimination rate constant and half-life for this patient can now be estimated from Eq. 23 and 28:

$$Kd = \frac{Cl}{Vd} \qquad \text{(Eq. 23)}$$

$$= \frac{38.75 \text{ L/day}}{235 \text{ L}}$$

$$= 0.165 \text{ day}^{-1}$$

$$t^{1/2} = \frac{(0.693)(Vd)}{Cl} \qquad \text{(Eq. 28)}$$

$$= \frac{(0.693)(235 \text{ L})}{38.75 \text{ L/day}}$$

$$= 4.2 \text{ days}$$

We now have the data necessary to answer the original question. The time required for her plasma level to fall from 4.0 ng/ml to 2.0 ng/ml (one-half the original level) is obviously one half-life, or 4.2 days.

In most situations the arithmetic is not this easy. In such cases the Kd and Eq. 24 can be used:

$$Kd = \frac{\ln\left(\frac{Cp_1}{Cp_2}\right)}{t} \qquad \text{(Eq. 24)}$$

$$t = \frac{\ln\left(\frac{Cp_1}{Cp_2}\right)}{Kd}$$

$$= \frac{\ln\left(\frac{4.0 \text{ ng/ml}}{2.0 \text{ ng/ml}}\right)}{0.165 \text{ days}^{-1}}$$

$$= \frac{\ln(2)}{0.165 \text{ days}^{-1}}$$

$$= 4.2 \text{ days}$$

8. Calculate a daily dose which will maintain this patient's average digoxin level at 2.0 ng/ml (mcg/L).

Using the clearance value of 38.75 L/day calculated from the patient's data, and assuming S, F and τ to be 1.0, 0.62 and 1 day respectively, the new maintenance dose could be estimated using Eq. 15:

$$\text{Maintenance Dose} = \frac{(Cl)(Cpss \text{ ave})(\tau)}{(S)(F)} \qquad \text{(Eq. 15)}$$

$$= \frac{(38.75 \text{ L/day})(2.0 \text{ mcg/L})(1 \text{ day})}{(1.0)(0.62)}$$

$$= \frac{77.5 \text{ mcg/day}}{0.62}$$

$$= 125 \text{ mcg/day } (0.125 \text{ mg/day})$$

Or, since we are assuming clearance and other factors to be constant, the previous maintenance dose could be adjusted proportionately to the desired change in steady state plasma level.

Therefore, if the new steady state level is to be one-half of the previous value, the new maintenance dose should be one-half the previous maintenance dose.

9. A patient who has been on the same dose of digoxin for 15 days comes in for follow-up and is found to be doing well clinically. A digoxin plasma level drawn on the morning of her visit is reported as 3.4 ng/ml. If the upper limit for therapeutic levels is 2.0 ng/ml, how can you account for the level being in the toxic range?

Since this level supposedly represents Cpss ave, one must evaluate each of the factors which may alter steady state. The relationship of each of these factors to steady state may be seen by studying Eq. 31:

$$\text{Cpss ave} = \frac{(S)(F)(\text{Dose}/\tau)}{Cl} \tag{Eq. 31}$$

a) (S)(F): the patient may be absorbing more than the average of 62%. (There are no salt forms of digoxin so S should be 1.0)
b) Dose: the patient may be taking more than the prescribed dose, although taking less than the prescribed dose is more common (45,64).
c) τ: the patient may be taking the proper dose more often than prescribed.
d) Cl: the patient's clearance or ability to eliminate the drug may be less than it was estimated to be.
e) Cpss ave: the assay could be in error, interfering substances may be present, or the plasma level may have been drawn during the distribution phase of the drug.

Plasma levels obtained during the distribution phase of digoxin are higher than anticipated because the drug is absorbed from the gastrointestinal tract faster than it is distributed into the tissues. Since the myocardium responds to digoxin as though it were in the tissue compartment (Vt), plasma levels obtained before distribution is complete do not correlate with pharmacologic effects of the drug (45,51). Most authors recommend that digoxin plasma levels be obtained just before the next dose is given, or that following a dose, a minimum of six hours be allowed to elapse before the sample is obtained (51). (See the discussion on Volume of Distribution at the beginning of this chapter.)

10. Outline a reasonable plan to determine the cause of this higher than predicted digoxin level.

a) Ask the patient whether the daily digoxin dose was taken before or after the blood sample was obtained.
b) Determine the patient's compliance. This is difficult but must be attempted through pill count or history.
c) Determine if any drugs interfered with the digoxin assay. Literature reports of interference by drugs having a steroid nucleus similar to that of digoxin are applicable only to the specific antibody and radioimmunoassay used in the particular report and may not apply to the specific assay used to determine the patient's digoxin plasma level. Therefore, the laboratory measuring the serum level would have to be contacted about the possibility of assay interference (67,68,69).
d) Radioisotopes such as those used in nuclear medicine can also influence radioimmunoassays (68). The patient's records should be reviewed for any recent diagnostic studies such as thyroid scan or cardiac studies that may have involved radioisotopes. Radioisotopes may cause a falsely elevated or depressed concentration depending on how the assay is performed. Again, the laboratory would have to be consulted if contamination with radioisotopes is a possibility.
e) Reschedule a second digoxin plasma level, but be certain that it is drawn a minimum of six hours after a dose. Preferably, obtain the sample in the morning *before* the daily dose is taken.
f) Evaluating the patient's Cl and F is difficult and costly because such evaluation would require hospitalization of the patient. It would only result in the obvious conclusion that the dose should be reduced if it was decided that, in fact, the level was too high. This approach would only be used

under the most unusual of circumstances. In addition, F could only increase from the assumed 0.65 to a maximum of 1.0 and could not by itself account for major changes in Cpss ave.

11. A patient receiving digoxin 0.375 mg/day for several months has a reported digoxin plasma concentration of 0.3 ng/ml and is noted to have poorly controlled congestive heart failure. What is the most probable explanation?

The answer to this question is essentially the same as that to Question 9, and the same factors should be considered.

$$\text{Cpss ave} = \frac{(S)(F)(Dose/\tau)}{Cl} \qquad \text{(Eq. 31)}$$

Certainly the patient should be asked if he is receiving the same brand of digoxin as before, and there is the possibility that he is one of the very rare patients who has a large metabolic clearance (73). The most likely explanation is noncompliance with the prescribed regimen (64).

12. In 1966, Doherty and Perkins (70) evaluated the kinetics of digoxin in hyperthyroid, hypothyroid and euthyroid patients. Fig. 2 is a representation of one of the graphs from this study. Using the graph, discuss the implications of thyroid disease on the loading dose, maintenance dose, and the time required to reach steady state, relative to the euthyroid state. Assume that the same Cpss ave is desired in all patients.

Loading dose: Since hypothyroid patients have higher plasma levels, they must have a decreased apparent volume of distribution. Therefore, a decrease in the loading doses would be appropriate. Hyperthyroid patients have lower plasma levels and would require larger loading doses for the same reasons.

Time to reach steady state: The slope of all the decay curves is the same. Therefore, the half-lives and elimination rate constants are equal, and the time required to reach steady state will be the same for hyperthyroid, hypothyroid and euthyroid patients receiving digoxin.

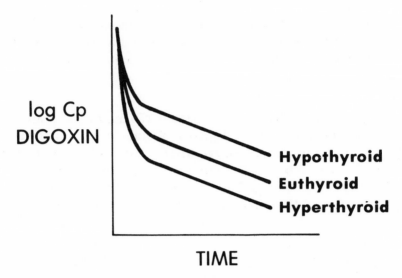

TIME

Fig. 2. Distribution and elimination of digoxin when administered by the intravenous route to hypothyroid, hyperthyroid and euthyroid patients (70).

Maintenance dose: Since Kd is the same in all patients, the
clearance and volume of distribution must both change by the
same proportion and in the same direction (see Eq. 23):

$$\frac{Cl_{(variable)}}{Vd_{(variable)}} = Kd_{(same\ in\ all\ patients\ studied)} \hspace{2cm} (Eq.\ 23)$$

Therefore, hypothyroid patients must have a decreased clearance as the volume of distribution is decreased. The reduction
in clearance would necessitate a reduction in maintenance
doses. Hyperthyroid patients must have an increased clearance
as the Vd is increased; therefore, an increase in maintenance
dose would be indicated if Cpss ave is to remain the same as for
euthyroid patients.

It is important to re-emphasize, however, that although Kd
and Vd were used to estimate clearance, Vd is an independent
variable which like Cl, is affected by thyroid disease. Since both
Cl and Vd were affected in the same direction, and to the same
degree, the half-life (and Kd) did not change.

Two recent studies (71,72) have examined the pharmacokinetics of digoxin in patients with thyroid disease. Both of these

suggest that the changes in the digoxin clearance may be the result of an increased glomerular filtration rate associated with hyperthyroidism. If this increased renal function *is* the primary factor responsible for the altered digoxin clearance observed in hyperthyroid patients, it would be possible to encounter such patients with *decreased* digoxin clearances if they also had intrinsic renal failure.

13. Do patients receiving hemodialysis require additional digoxin following dialysis?

No. The dialysis clearance for digoxin is only 10 ml/min. Therefore, less than 3% of the amount in the body is removed during hemodialysis (74). This dialysis clearance of 10 ml/min may seem significant when compared to the metabolic clearance of 23 ml/min for patients with congestive heart failure (6), but the dialysis takes place for only 6 hours every few days, while the metabolic clearance is continuing to remove drug 24 hours a day 7 days a week, making the dialysis clearance comparatively minor.

However, dialysis can induce digitalis toxicity because of alterations in serum electrolytes and acid-base balance. For example, a high serum potassium which is protecting a patient from digitalis toxicity may be decreased during dialysis, resulting in signs of toxicity during or just following dialysis.

14. A patient receiving digoxin 0.25 mg/day for atrial fibrillation is about to be started on quinidine. What are your considerations?

Recent studies have indicated that patients receiving digoxin have a rapid and sustained rise in the serum digoxin concentration following the addition of quinidine (75,76). The change in digoxin concentration occurs within a few days (75) and the final digoxin concentration is doubled. Many of the patients develop signs of digitalis toxicity which subside when the dose and plasma concentrations are adjusted.

The rapid and sustained changes in digoxin concentrations suggest that both the volume of distribution and clearance for digoxin are reduced by the addition of quinidine. Patients receiving digoxin who are to begin quinidine therapy should be monitored very closely for the first 7 to 14 days following the addition of quinidine. If it is clinically appropriate one may consider empirically reducing the digoxin dose by half, obtaining digoxin levels and making further adjustments as necessary. These are only guidelines, however, as the full implications of the quinidine-digoxin interaction have not been determined (226,227,228).

3

Lidocaine

Lidocaine is an antiarrhythmic agent which is used acutely for the treatment of severe ventricular arrhythmias. Lidocaine has poor oral bioavailability, is almost exclusively metabolized by the liver, and has a relatively short duration of action. For these reasons, one or more intravenous boluses of 1–2 mg/kg are administered initially to achieve an immediate response, followed by an infusion of 1–4 mg/min to maintain the therapeutic effect. Lidocaine has a narrow therapeutic index and toxic effects are generally dose related. Further, concurrent conditions such as congestive heart failure and liver dysfunction may alter the kinetics of lidocaine and, therefore, expected therapeutic responses to usual doses. The application of pharmacokinetic principles to the individualization of lidocaine dosing can be invaluable.

Therapeutic and Toxic Plasma Levels

Lidocaine plasma concentrations of 1 to 5 mcg/ml (mg/L) are usually associated with therapeutic control of ventricular arrhythmias (130,131,132). Minor CNS side effects of dizziness, mental confusion and blurred vision can be observed in patients with plasma concentrations as low as 3 to 5 mcg/ml. Seizures occasionally occur with plasma concentrations as low as 6 mcg/ml, but usually they are associated with concentrations exceeding 9 mcg/ml (22,48,130,131,132). Lidocaine does not usually cause hemodynamic changes, but hypotension associated with myocardial depression has been observed in a patient whose plasma lidocaine concentration was 5.3 mcg/ml (133). In addition, there are reports of sinus arrest following rapid intravenous injection (138).

Volume of Distribution

The distribution of lidocaine following an intravenous bolus can be described by a two compartment body model (see Part One, Fig.

93

KEY PARAMETERS					
Therapeutic Plasma Concentrations	1–5 mcg/ml (mg/L)				
	Vi	Vd	$\alpha t\frac{1}{2}$	$\beta t\frac{1}{2}$	Cl
Normal	0.5 L/kg	1.3 L/kg	8 min	100 min	10 ml/min/kg
CHF	0.3 L/kg	0.88 L/kg	8 min	100 min	6 ml/min/kg
Cirrhosis	0.61 L/kg	2.3 L/kg	8 min	300 min	6 ml/min/kg

9). The initial volume of distribution (Vi) appears to be about 0.5 L/kg and the final volume following distribution (Vd) is about 1.3 L/kg (22,48). Unlike digoxin, the myocardium responds as though it were located in the initial volume, Vi. Therefore, the dose of each *bolus* injection of lidocaine should be based on Vi and not Vd. However, plasma concentrations resulting from each bolus injection will fall as the drug distributes into the larger final volume of distribution. Therefore, the *total* loading dose should be calculated using the final volume of distribution (Vd).

In *congestive heart failure (CHF)*, both volumes of distribution for lidocaine are decreased: Vi is 0.3 L/kg and Vd is 0.88 L/kg. Both the total loading dose and the individual bolus injections should be reduced in patients with congestive heart failure. In *chronic liver disease*, on the other hand, both volumes of distribution are increased: Vi is 0.61 L/kg and Vd is 2.3 L/kg. Thus, slightly larger loading doses may be required in these patients. Renal failure does not appear to alter the distribution of lidocaine. (48)

Clearance

Lidocaine has a high hepatic extraction ratio. Its clearance of 10 ml/min/kg (700 ml/min/70 kg) approximates plasma flow to the liver (7,19,48). Less than 5% is cleared by the renal route. Following an oral dose, almost all of the drug is metabolized before reaching the systemic circulation; therefore, parenteral administration is required.

Congestive heart failure and *hepatic cirrhosis* decrease the clearance of lidocaine to about 6 ml/kg/min, making a 40% reduction in the maintenance infusion appropriate for patients with these diseases (48,140,141). Since the drug is not cleared by the renal route, no dose adjustment is required for patients with diminished renal function.

Lidocaine is broken down into two major metabolites: monoethylglycinexylidine (MEGX) and glycinexylidide (GX). MEGX appears to have activity similar to lidocaine. It is cleared by metabolism and therefore does not accumulate in renal failure. However, approximately 50% of GX is cleared by the renal route and it, therefore, accumulates in patients with diminished renal function (135). GX is less active than lidocaine and does not contribute to its therapeutic effect. The only known side effects of GX are headache and impaired mental performance which occur at plasma concentrations greater than 1.0 mg/L (135). More serious toxicities have not been observed in patients with GX levels as high as 9 mg/L (136).

Half-life

The *distribution half-life* ($\alpha t\frac{1}{2}$) of 8 minutes does not appear to be altered by heart failure, hepatic disease or renal failure.

The *elimination half-life* ($\beta t\frac{1}{2}$) of lidocaine is a function of its volume of distribution and clearance:

$$t\frac{1}{2} = \frac{(0.693)(Vd)}{Cl} \qquad \text{(Eq. 28)}$$

The usual elimination half-life for lidocaine is about 100 minutes (48). It is similar for patients with congestive heart failure because in these individuals both the volume of distribution and the clearance are reduced to a similar extent.

Patients with liver disease have a lidocaine β half-life of about 300 minutes due to an increased volume of distribution and decreased clearance (134). An elimination half-life of 200 minutes has recently been observed in healthy subjects following infusions lasting longer than 24 hours (134).

1. P.M., a 55-year-old 70 kg male, was admitted to the coronary care unit with a diagnosis of heart failure, probable myocardial infarction, and premature ventricular con-

tractions. **Calculate a loading dose of lidocaine for this patient which should achieve an immediate response. At what rate should this dose be administered?**

The loading dose which will be given as the initial bolus is calculated using Eq. 10. However, because lidocaine distribution follows a two compartment model with the myocardium responding as though it were in the initial compartment, Vd in Eq. 10 should be replaced with Vi (see the discussion of Volume of Distribution at the beginning of this chapter). The Vi for a patient with congestive heart failure is 0.3 L/kg or 21 L for this 70 kg male (48). S and F are assumed to be 1.0 for lidocaine. If it is assumed that to avoid toxicity peak levels should not exceed 3 mcg/ml (mg/L), the appropriate bolus dose would be 63 mg:

$$\text{Loading Dose} = \frac{(Vd)(Cp)}{(S)(F)} \qquad \text{(Eq. 10)}$$

$$\begin{aligned}\text{Dose for} \\ \text{Lidocaine} \\ \text{Bolus}\end{aligned} = \frac{(Vi)(Cp)}{(S)(F)}$$

$$= \frac{(21\ L)(3\ mg/L)}{(1.0)(1.0)}$$

$$= 63\ mg$$

This bolus dose of 63 mg is essentially the same as the usually recommended dose of 1 to 2 mg/kg (137) and should be given by slow IV push (25 to 50 mg/minute).

2. Calculate a maintenance infusion rate for this patient which will achieve a steady state plasma lidocaine concentration of 2 mcg/ml.

The maintenance dose can be calculated from Eq. 15. If it is assumed that a steady state concentration of 2 mcg/ml is desired and if τ is assumed to be one minute, Cl to be 420 ml/min (6 ml/min/kg for a patient in congestive heart failure), and S and F are 1.0, the maintenance dose would be calculated as follows:

$$\text{Maintenance Dose} = \frac{(Cl)(Cpss\ ave)(\tau)}{(S)(F)} \qquad \text{(Eq. 15)}$$

$$= \frac{(420\ ml/min)(2\ mcg/ml)(1\ min)}{(1.0)(1.0)}$$

= 840 mcg/min

= 0.84 mg/min

This calculated infusion is compatible with the frequently recommended 1 to 4 mg/minute infusion rates (137), considering the conservative target steady state level of 2 mcg/ml and the expected decrease in clearance in a patient with congestive heart failure.

Note: The assumed clearance value of 6 ml/kg/min for heart failure is an average value. Zito and Reid have developed a scaling procedure in which the recommended lidocaine infusion rate is based upon the degree of heart failure. The following table is adapted from their data (139):

Clinical Class	Symptoms	Apparent Lidocaine Clearance, ml/min/kg
I	No heart failure	14.5
II	S-3 gallop and basilar pulmonary rales	5
III	Pulmonary edema	
IV	Cardiogenic shock	2.1

3. P.M.'s PVC's were controlled by the 63 mg bolus dose of lidocaine and an infusion of 1 mg/minute was begun. Fifteen minutes later, PVC's were again noted. Explain. What would be an appropriate course of action?

The distribution half-life of lidocaine is about 8 minutes and the elimination half-life is 1.5 to 2 hours. Since three to four elimination half-lives (approximately 6 hours) must pass before steady state plasma levels resulting from the infusion can be evaluated, it is most likely that the recurrence of the PVC's 15 minutes after the bolus dose represents a declining plasma concentration due to distribution rather than a maintenance dose which is too low. Furthermore, it is likely that even after starting the maintenance infusion, an additional bolus injection will be required because the predicted average steady state lidocaine concentration after distribution is 1 mg/L. This concentration is determined by using the final volume of distribution (Vd) in a rearranged version of Eq. 10:

$$\text{Loading Dose} = \frac{(Vd)(Cp)}{(S)(F)} \qquad\qquad \text{(Eq. 10)}$$

$$Cp^0 = \frac{(S)(F)(Dose)}{Vd} \qquad\qquad \text{(Eq. 40)}$$

$$= \frac{(1)(1)(63 \text{ mg})}{62 \text{ L}}$$

$$= 1 \text{ mg/L}$$

For these reasons it would be most rational to administer a second bolus dose rather than change the infusion rate. In practice, the second or third bolus doses are reduced by one-half to avoid excessive accumulation. In addition, some clinicians will increase the maintenance infusion for 20 to 30 minutes to allow for more rapid accumulation and then reduce the infusion back to the original rate.

If the PVC's had occurred several hours after starting the infusion, the most rational approach would have been to give a small bolus dose sufficient to increase the plasma concentration in the initial volume of distribution by 2 or 3 mg/L and to increase the infusion rate as well.

4. B.P., a 65-year-old patient weighing 70 kg, was admitted for hepatic encephalopathy and cirrhosis. On the fourth hospital day he developed ventricular arrhythmias and lidocaine was ordered. Calculate a loading dose and a maintenance infusion which will achieve a steady state lidocaine level of 2 mcg/ml (mg/L).

In patients with chronic liver disease the following pharmacokinetic parameters for lidocaine would be expected (48):

Vi   43 L (0.61 L/kg)
Vd 161 L (2.3 L/kg)
Cl   420 ml/min or 25.2 L/hr (6 ml/kg/min)

As in Question 1, the initial bolus can be calculated from Eq. 10, replacing Vd with Vi. Assuming a maximum level of 3 mg/L (mcg/ml) is desired, the initial bolus should be 129 mg:

$$\text{Loading Dose} = \frac{(Vi)(Cp)}{(S)(F)} \qquad \text{(Eq. 10)}$$

$$= \frac{(43 \text{ L})(3 \text{ mg/L})}{(1)(1)}$$

$$= 129 \text{ mg}$$

Again, this dose should be given no more rapidly than 25 to 50 mg/minute.

After final distribution, this dose of 129 mg should result in a plasma level of 0.8 mg/L:

$$Cp^0 = \frac{(S)(F)(Dose)}{Vd} \qquad \text{(Eq. 40)}$$

$$= \frac{(1)(1)(129 \text{ mg})}{161 \text{ L}}$$

$$= 0.8 \text{ mg/L}$$

Since this anticipated plasma concentration is rather low, it is likely that an additional bolus will be required. To avoid excessive accumulation, about half the original dose is usually given when additional bolus doses are required.

The maintenance infusion can be calculated from Eq. 15, using the expected clearance of 420 ml/min:

$$\text{Maintenance Dose} = \frac{(Cl)(Cpss \text{ ave})(\tau)}{(S)(F)} \qquad \text{(Eq. 15)}$$

$$= \frac{(420 \text{ ml/min})(2 \text{ mcg/ml})(1 \text{ min})}{(1)(1)}$$

$$= 840 \text{ mcg/min}$$

$$= 0.84 \text{ mg/min}$$

Thus, a maintenance infusion of 0.84 mg/hour should achieve a steady state plasma concentration of 2 mcg/ml.

5. Eighteen hours after starting the infusion, B.P. appears to be more confused than usual, and it is not clear whether his present condition is secondary to hepatic encephalopathy or lidocaine. Is it possible that the lidocaine is still accumulating and causing the impaired mental state?

The expected half-life for lidocaine in this patient can be calculated from his assumed lidocaine Cl and Vd:

$$t\tfrac{1}{2} = \frac{(0.693)(Vd)}{Cl} \qquad \text{(Eq. 28)}$$

$$= \frac{(0.693)(161 \text{ L})}{25.2 \text{ L/hr}}$$

$$= 4.42 \text{ hrs}$$

This calculated value of 4.4 hours is reasonably close to the value of 4.9 hours which is reported in the literature for patients with hepatic failure (48). Since the expected half-life for lidocaine in this patient is 4 to 5 hours, steady state levels may not have been achieved after 18 hours and his lidocaine levels may still be rising. (See Part One, section on Half-Life). Furthermore, even in healthy subjects, the half-life of lidocaine appears to increase after prolonged infusions (134,140,141); after receiving a constant infusion for 24 hours, the lidocaine concentration in many patients may still be slowly rising.

4

Procainamide

Procainamide is used in the treatment of ventricular tachyar-rhythmias and is administered orally, intramuscularly, and intra-venously. A loading dose of approximately 1000 mg is generally followed by maintenance doses of 250 to 500 mg every 3 to 4 hours. Because its short half-life requires frequent administration and because long-term administration is frequently associated with immunologic reactions, the use of procainamide is often lim-ited to the hospital setting.

Pharmacokinetic predictions are complicated by the fact that procainamide is metabolized to an active metabolite, N-acetylpro-cainamide (NAPA), which is an antiarrhythmic in its own right. Therefore, administration of procainamide requires consideration of two drugs acting in tandem.

PROCAINAMIDE

Therapeutic and Toxic Plasma Concentrations

Plasma procainamide concentrations of 4 to 8 mcg/ml (mg/L) are usually considered therapeutic (77,78). Minor toxicities such as GI disturbances, weakness, mild hypotension, and a 10 to 30% pro-longation in the P-R, Q-T, or QRS intervals are not usually seen with plasma concentrations below 8 mcg/ml but occur in as many as 30% of patients with plasma concentrations of 12 to 16 mcg/ml (78). Severe toxicities such as hypotension, conduction disturb-ances, or ventricular arrhythmias occur in about 40% of patients with plasma concentrations of 16 mcg/ml or greater (78).

Bioavailability

The bioavailability of orally administered procainamide is ap-proximately 85% (F = 0.85) (182). Absorption is usually rapid,

101

```
┌─────────────────────────────────────────────────────────────────┐
│                         KEY PARAMETERS                            │
│                                                                   │
│   Therapeutic Concentrations          4–8 mcg/ml                  │
│   Bioavailability (F)                 0.85                        │
│   Vdᵃ                                 2 L/kg                      │
│   Clᵇ                                 550 ml/min (33 L/hr)        │
│   αt½                                 5 min                       │
│   βt½ᶜ                                ≈ 3 hr                      │
│   S (HCl salt)                        0.87                        │
│   ─────────                                                       │
│   ᵃ Decreased by 25% in patient with low cardiac output.         │
│   ᵇ 50% metabolized (15 to 30% of the total clearance to NAPA, an active │
│     metabolite). 50% cleared renally. Reduced in severe congestive heart fail- │
│     ure.                                                          │
│   ᶜ 5 hours in patients with congestive heart failure.           │
└─────────────────────────────────────────────────────────────────┘
```

KEY PARAMETERS	
Therapeutic Concentrations	4–8 mcg/ml
Bioavailability (F)	0.85
Vd[a]	2 L/kg
Cl[b]	550 ml/min (33 L/hr)
$\alpha t\frac{1}{2}$	5 min
$\beta t\frac{1}{2}$[c]	≈ 3 hr
S (HCl salt)	0.87

[a] Decreased by 25% in patient with low cardiac output.
[b] 50% metabolized (15 to 30% of the total clearance to NAPA, an active metabolite). 50% cleared renally. Reduced in severe congestive heart failure.
[c] 5 hours in patients with congestive heart failure.

and peak plasma concentrations occur approximately one hour after administration. However, considerable variation in absorption occurs among individuals (182), and absorption can be very slow and incomplete in patients with congestive heart failure (77).

Volume of Distribution

The volume of distribution of procainamide is approximately 2 L/kg (78,79,181). This volume is unchanged by renal failure (181) but is decreased by about 25% in patients with decreased cardiac output (78).

Like lidocaine, procainamide distributes into an initial volume of distribution (Vi) (77,78,183). This initial volume is approximately one-third the volume of distribution that is observed after the drug has distributed into and equilibrated with the tissue volume of distribution (77,181,183). Since the myocardium responds as though it were located in the initial volume of distribution, loading doses (which are calculated on the basis of Vd) should be given in increments small enough to avoid excessive plasma concentrations in Vi.

Clearance

The clearance of procainamide in an average 70 kg patient with reasonably good renal function is about 550 ml/min; one-half of the drug is cleared by metabolism and one-half is cleared renally

(77). This clearance is reduced in patients with significant congestive heart failure (78). Although subjects with excellent renal
function and cardiac output may have procainamide clearances of
600 to 800 ml/min (182,183,185), a value of 550 ml/min is more
appropriately used in the clinical setting.

Half-life

The apparent distribution half-life ($\alpha t\frac{1}{2}$) is about 5 minutes
(78,182,183). The elimination half-life ($\beta t\frac{1}{2}$) of procainamide is a
function of its volume of distribution and clearance:

$$t\frac{1}{2} = \frac{(0.693)(Vd)}{Cl} \qquad \text{(Eq. 28)}$$

Thus, for a patient with a Vd of 140 L (2 L/kg $\times$ 70 kg) and a
clearance of 33 L/hr (550 ml/min $\times$ 60 min/hr $\div$ 1000 ml/L), the
expected elimination half-life would be approximately 3 hours:

$$t\frac{1}{2} = \frac{(0.093)(140\ L)}{33\ L/hr}$$

$$\approx 3\ \text{hours}$$

Because the half-life is so short, frequent dosing will be necessary
prior to the accumulation of therapeutic plasma concentrations of
the active metabolite, NAPA. In patients with congestive heart
failure the half-life of procainamide is increased to approximately
5 hours (186).

NAPA

Therapeutic and Toxic Plasma Concentrations

The exact relationship between plasma N-acetylprocainamide
(NAPA) concentrations and antiarrhythmic activity has not been
clearly established. Its activity has been observed to be similar to
that of procainamide when equal plasma concentrations are compared (179,187,190). However, others have found that plasma concentrations of approximately 10 to 20 mcg/ml are required for
suppression of premature ventricular contractions (178,180). It
has been suggested that very little additional antiarrhythmic ef-

fects are seen when NAPA concentrations exceed 30 mcg/ml (180). Interestingly, when the therapeutic levels of 4–8 mcg/ml for procainamide were established (77,78), NAPA concentrations were not considered. Since plasma NAPA concentrations are approximately equal to procainamide concentrations in many patients (188,189), the total concentration of procainamide plus NAPA may have been in the range of 8 to 16 mcg/ml in the patients used to establish the therapeutic concentrations of procainamide.

Evidence from animal studies suggests that NAPA may be less toxic than procainamide (179). Significant cardiac toxicity has not been observed with NAPA concentrations as high as 40 mcg/ml (180). In addition, the development of systemic lupus erythematosus may be less likely with NAPA than procainamide (190).

NAPA Production

The rate of NAPA production is dependent upon the rate of N-acetylation of procainamide which in turn is genetically determined. About 50% of Blacks and Caucasians are rapid acetylators, and approximately 80 to 90% of Asians are rapid acetylators. Rapid acetylators convert approximately 30% of an administered dose of procainamide to NAPA, while slow acetylators convert about 15% (29). Since total procainamide clearance is approximately 550 ml/min (77), or 33 L/hr/70 kg, the clearance of procainamide to NAPA would be expected to be about 10 L/hr (33 L/hr × 0.30) for a 70 kg rapid acetylator and about 5 L/hr (33 L/hr × 0.15) for a 70 kg slow acetylator. These values are reasonably close to clearance values that have been reported (181).

Volume of Distribution

The volume of distribution (Vd) of NAPA appears to be about 1.5 L/kg (193,194).

Clearance

NAPA appears to have a total clearance of about 3.2 ml/min/kg, or 13 L/hr/70 kg (193). About 80 to 85% of this clearance occurs renally, indicating that the renal clearance of NAPA is approximately 10.5 L/hr/70 kg and the metabolic clearance is approximately 2.4 L/hr/70 kg (193).

Half-life

The usual half-life of NAPA in patients with normal renal function is approximately 6 hours, but the half-life may increase to 30 hours or more in patients with poor renal function (181,185).

1. **A.L., a 62-year-old 70 kg man, was admitted to the coronary care unit with a diagnosis of acute myocardial infarction (AMI). He has a history of mild chronic renal failure and a serum creatinine of 1.3 mg/dl with a creatinine clearance of 50 ml/min. A.L. developed premature ventricular contractions (PVC's) which did not respond to lidocaine. Calculate a parenteral loading dose of procainamide designed to achieve a plasma concentration of 8 mcg/ml (mg/L).**

To calculate the total loading dose required to achieve a procainamide level of 8 mcg/ml, the volume of distribution must be estimated. Assuming A.L. does not have significant heart failure, the expected volume of distribution would be 140 L (2 L/kg). Using Eq. 10 and assuming F to be 1.0 for parenteral administration and S to be 0.87 for the hydrochloride salt, the loading dose of procainamide would be:

$$\text{Loading Dose} = \frac{(Vd)(Cp)}{(S)(F)} \quad \text{(Eq. 10)}$$

$$= \frac{(140 \text{ L})(8 \text{ mg/L})}{(0.87)(1.0)}$$

$$= 1287 \text{ mg, or about } 1300 \text{ mg}$$

This calculated loading dose is reasonably close to the usual loading dose of 1000 mg (184). If the patient had had congestive heart failure, the volume of distribution, and therefore the loading dose, would have been decreased by about 25% (78).

2. **If the loading dose of 1300 mg is to be given intravenously, how should it be administered?**

Since procainamide is administered into an initial volume of distribution (Vi) (77,78,183) and the myocardium responds as though it were located in this initial volume (78,183,184), the loading dose should be given in divided doses. If the entire loading dose were given as a single bolus, the initial plasma concentrations would greatly exceed the desired 8 mg/L. If the apparent initial volume of distribution is about one-third the total Vd, as much as one-third of the loading dose may be given as the first bolus. In this case, 300 to 400 could be administered initially followed by doses of 150 to 200 mg (one-half the original dose) every 5 minutes. Since the apparent distribution half-life is about 5 minutes (78,183), each of the doses should be separated by at least 5 minutes to avoid accumulation in Vi. In most clinical situations 100 mg is given every 5 minutes until the arrhythmia is abolished or the total loading dose is administered (184). Others have recommended infusing the total loading dose at a rate of 16 mg/minute to achieve therapeutic concentrations relatively rapidly while avoiding excessive accumulation in the first compartment (185). Whatever method is employed, the patient should be closely monitored for side effects such as hypotension and rhythm disturbances that may be procainamide-related.

3. Calculate an infusion rate in mg/min which will maintain an average plasma procainamide concentration of 6 mcg/ml (mg/L) for A.L., the patient described in Question 1.

Since clearance is the determinant of the maintenance dose, this parameter must be estimated before the infusion rate can be calculated. In an average 70 kg patient with reasonably good renal function, procainamide appears to have a plasma clearance of approximately 550 ml/min. Since 50% is cleared metabolically and 50% is cleared renally, the metabolic and renal clearance are 275 ml/min each. A.L.'s renal clearance of procainamide will be decreased since his creatinine clearance of 50 ml/min represents only half of the usual value of approximately 100 ml/min. Eq. 21 can be used to estimate his procainamide clearance:

$$\text{Cl}_{\text{adjusted}} = \frac{\text{Cl}_m + (\text{Cl}_r \times \text{Fraction of Normal Renal}}{\text{Function Remaining})} \qquad \text{(Eq. 21)}$$

$$= 275 \text{ ml/min} + (275 \text{ ml/min} \times 0.5)$$

$$= 275 \text{ ml/min} + 137.5 \text{ ml/min}$$

$$= 412.5 \text{ ml/min}$$

$$= \frac{412.5 \text{ ml/min} \times 60 \text{ min/hr}}{1000 \text{ ml/L}}$$

$$= 24.75 \text{ L/hr}$$

Using this clearance and the desired average steady state concentration, Eq. 15 can be used to calculate the maintenance dose. Since procainamide is administered as the HCl salt, S is 0.87, F is 1.0 for the intravenous route, and τ should be one hour if clearance is stated in L/hr or one minute if clearance is expressed as ml/min.

$$\text{Maintenance Dose} = \frac{(\text{Cl})(\text{Cpss ave})(\tau)}{(\text{S})(\text{F})} \qquad \text{(Eq. 15)}$$

$$= \frac{(24.75 \text{ L/hr})(6 \text{ mg/L})(1 \text{ hr})}{(0.87)(1.0)}$$

$$= 170.6 \text{ mg/hr}$$

4. A.B. is a 70 kg patient who has been receiving a constant procainamide infusion of 100 mg/hr which has resulted in a steady state plasma procainamide concentration of 5 mcg/ml. His creatinine clearance is 30 ml/min. Calculate an oral dosing regimen that will maintain his plasma procainamide concentration between 4 and 8 mcg/ml (mg/L).

Because the trough concentrations are to be no less than half of the peak levels, the dosing interval cannot be longer than the half-life. The half-life of procainamide in this patient can be estimated if the Vd and clearance are known:

$$t\tfrac{1}{2} = \frac{(0.693)(\text{Vd})}{\text{Cl}} \qquad \text{(Eq. 28)}$$

Assuming A.B. does not have significant congestive heart failure, the average volume of distribution of 140 L (2 L/kg) can be used. However, his creatinine clearance indicates that his renal clearance of procainamide will be less than normal. The latter can be determined from his dosing history and reported steady state plasma concentration using Eq. 14 (assuming S to be 0.87 and F to be 1.0):

$$Cl = \frac{(S)(F)(Dose/\tau)}{Cpss\ ave} \qquad\qquad (Eq.\ 14)$$

$$= \frac{(0.87)(1.0)(100\ mg/hr)}{5\ mg/L}$$

$$= \frac{87\ mg/hr}{5\ mg/L}$$

$$= 17.4\ L/hr$$

Using this clearance, the half-life of procainamide in this patient can now be calculated:

$$t\tfrac{1}{2} = \frac{(0.693)(Vd)}{Cl} \qquad\qquad (Eq.\ 28)$$

$$= \frac{(0.693)(140\ L)}{17.4\ L/hr}$$

$$= 5.6\ hrs$$

The dosing interval should be no longer than 5.6 hours.

The oral maintenance dose can be calculated by first selecting a convenient dosing interval which is less than 5.6 hours (for example, 4 hours); then, Eq. 15 can be used to calculate the maintenance dose. The average steady state concentration in this equation can be assumed to be about half-way between the maximum and minimum concentrations, or in this case 6 mg/L. If the bioavailability for procainamide is assumed to be 85% (F = 0.85) (182) and S is 0.87 for the hydrochloride salt, the maintenance dose will be 565 mg every 4 hours:

$$Maintenance\ Dose = \frac{(Cl)(Cpss\ ave)(\tau)}{(S)(F)} \qquad\qquad (Eq.\ 15)$$

$$= \frac{(17.4\ L/hr)(6\ mg/L)(4\ hr)}{(0.87)(0.85)}$$

$$= \frac{417.6\ mg}{0.739}$$

$$= 565\ mg$$

Since procainamide is available in 250, 375 and 500 mg dosage forms, a dose of 500 mg every 4 hours might be selected. The expected peak and trough concentrations could be calculated using Equations 36 and 38.

$$\text{Cpss max} = \frac{\dfrac{(S)(F)(Dose)}{Vd}}{1 - e^{-Kd\tau}} \qquad \text{(Eq. 36)}$$

$$\text{Cpss min} = (\text{Cpss max})(e^{-Kd\tau}) \qquad \text{(Eq. 38)}$$

To solve the above equations, Kd must first be calculated. The elimination rate constant can be determined from the half-life (5.6 hours) by rearranging Eq. 27:

$$t\tfrac{1}{2} = \frac{0.693}{Kd} \qquad \text{(Eq. 27)}$$

$$Kd = \frac{0.693}{t\tfrac{1}{2}}$$

$$= \frac{0.693}{5.6 \text{ hr}}$$

$$= 0.124 \text{ hr}^{-1}$$

Then, a Cpss max of 6.77 mg/L can be calculated:

$$\text{Cpss max} = \frac{\dfrac{(S)(F)(Dose)}{Vd}}{1 - e^{-Kd\tau}} \qquad \text{(Eq. 36)}$$

$$= \frac{(0.87)(0.85)(500 \text{ mg})/140 \text{ L}}{1 - e^{-(0.124/hr)(4 \text{ hr})}}$$

$$= \frac{369.75 \text{ mg}/140 \text{ L}}{1 - e^{-0.496}}$$

$$= \frac{2.64 \text{ mg/L}}{1 - 0.61}$$

$$= \frac{2.64 \text{ mg/L}}{0.39}$$

$$= 6.77 \text{ mg/L}$$

Once Cpss max is known, a Cpss min of 4.13 mg/L can be calculated:

$$\text{Cpss min} = (\text{Cpss max})(e^{-K_d\tau}) \qquad \text{(Eq. 38)}$$

$$= (6.77 \text{ mg/L})(e^{-(0.124/hr)(4 \text{ hr})})$$

$$= (6.77 \text{ mg/L})(e^{-0.496})$$

$$= (6.77 \text{ mg/L})(0.61)$$

$$= 4.13 \text{ mg/L}$$

The predicted peak and trough plasma concentrations of 6.77 mg/L and 4.13 mg/L respectively were based upon the assumption that absorption occurs rapidly. The dampening effect of absorption will produce peak concentrations that are slightly lower and trough concentrations that are slightly higher than predicted by the IV bolus model. One should recall that absorption rates vary considerably among patients (182), especially those with congestive heart failure (77).

5. A.B., who was described in the previous question, has a steady state plasma procainamide concentration of 5 mcg/ml. Estimate his plasma NAPA concentration.

The steady state NAPA concentration can be determined from Eq. 31 once the necessary parameters are derived.

$$\text{Cpss ave} = \frac{(S)(F)(\text{Dose}/\tau)}{Cl} \qquad \text{(Eq. 31)}$$

In this case it can be assumed that S and F are 1.0, since NAPA is produced directly from plasma procainamide. The rate of NAPA production (Dose/τ) can be calculated by multiplying the average steady state procainamide concentration by the clearance of procainamide to NAPA. If the patient is phenotypically a rapid acetylator, the clearance to NAPA would be about 10 L/hr/70 kg. If he is a slow acetylator, it would be 5 L/hr/70 kg. Assuming he is a rapid acetylator, his rate of NAPA production would be:

$$\text{Rate of Conversion to NAPA} = (\text{Cpss ave})(Cl_{\text{to NAPA}})$$

$$= (5 \text{ mg/L})(10 \text{ L/hr})$$

$$= 50 \text{ mg/hr}$$

This approach assumes that the molecular weight of procainamide and NAPA are similar and each milligram of procainamide converted to NAPA represents a milligram of NAPA. Once the rate of NAPA production (which is essentially the infusion rate of NAPA) and the clearance for NAPA are known, the average steady state plasma concentration can be calculated from Eq. 31. Since the patient has reduced renal function, his NAPA clearance will be reduced. This reduced clearance can be estimated using Eq. 21:

$$Cl_{adjusted} = \frac{Cl_m + (Cl_r \times \text{Fraction of Normal Renal}}{\text{Function Remaining})} \quad \text{(Eq. 21)}$$

If the usual metabolic clearance of NAPA is 2.4 L/hr/70 kg, the usual renal clearance is 10.5 L/hr/70 kg, and the fraction of renal function remaining is 0.3 (30 ml/min ÷ 100 ml/min), the adjusted clearance for NAPA in this 70 kg patient would be:

$$Cl_{adjusted} = 2.4 \text{ L/hr} + (10.5 \text{ L/hr} \times 0.3)$$
$$= 2.4 \text{ L/hr} + 3.15 \text{ L/hr}$$
$$= 5.55 \text{ L/hr}$$

Eq. 31 can now be used to predict the steady state plasma concentration of NAPA:

$$\text{Cpss ave} = \frac{(S)(F)(Dose/\tau)}{Cl} \quad \text{(Eq. 31)}$$
$$= \frac{(1)(1)(50 \text{ mg/hr})}{5.55 \text{ L/hr}}$$
$$= 9 \text{ mg/L}$$

6. What is the clinical significance of plasma NAPA concentrations? How might they alter the clinical use of procainamide and interpretation of plasma procainamide concentrations?

Therapeutic plasma concentrations of procainamide were established before it was known that NAPA could be contributing to the therapeutic and possibly toxic effects of procainamide. The ratio of NAPA to procainamide concentrations is primarily a function of phenotype and renal function. Patients with poor renal function who are rapid acetylators will have the highest ratios of NAPA to procainamide concentrations.

Patients with high NAPA to procainamide ratios may experience therapeutic effects even when average or trough concentrations of procainamide are below those usually associated with antiarrhythmic control. The longer half-life of NAPA may also explain why many patients, especially those with renal failure, are well controlled on procainamide even though the dosing intervals are longer than 4 to 5 hours; NAPA concentrations change relatively little when the procainamide dosing interval is 6 hours.

Also, if NAPA is contributing to the antiarrhythmic effect, the full efficacy of a procainamide dosing regimen cannot be evaluated until NAPA concentrations have reached steady state. In patients with renal failure who have a NAPA half-life of 30 hours or longer, five days or more may be required before steady state NAPA concentrations are attained and maximal antiarrhythmic effects are observed. A similar situation will be encountered when procainamide is discontinued in patients with poor renal function. Within 24 to 36 hours after discontinuing the drug, procainamide levels will essentially be zero; however, one cannot ascertain whether or not the patient can be maintained without procainamide until several more days have elapsed and NAPA levels have declined substantially.

To illustrate these principles, this information can be applied to A.B., the patient described in the previous two questions. Eq. 28 can be used to calculate the half-life for NAPA if a volume of distribution of 105 L (1.5 L/kg × 70 kg) and a clearance of 5.55 L/hr previously calculated in Question 5 are used:

$$t\frac{1}{2} = \frac{(0.693)(Vd)}{Cl} \qquad \text{(Eq. 28)}$$

$$= \frac{(0.693)(105 \text{ L})}{5.55 \text{ L/hr}}$$

$$= 13.1 \text{ hours}$$

To determine how long it will take to observe maximal antiarrhythmic effects of the procainamide, one must also consider the time required to achieve steady state procainamide concentrations since maximum NAPA production does not occur until steady state procainamide levels are attained. The procainamide levels will plateau 15 hours after beginning the initial infusion (3 hours × 5 half-lives). Therefore, more than three days will be required (15 hours + 13.1 hours × 5 half-lives) before A.B. achieves steady state NAPA concentrations and experiences the maximum effects of his procainamide dosage regimen. Similarly, upon cessation of therapy his procainamide levels should be approaching zero after 15 hours (assuming no continued absorption from his GI tract), but 15 hours is not much longer than one NAPA half-life so his NAPA concentrations at this time will be about one-half of their steady state value (9.0 mcg/ml ÷ 2 = 4.5 mcg/ml). Therefore, it is possible that therapeutic effects could persist even in the absence of measurable plasma procainamide concentrations.

5

Quinidine

Quinidine is used in the treatment of atrial fibrillation and other cardiac arrhythmias. It is administered orally as the sulfate, gluconate or polygalacturonate salts and by intravenous infusions prepared from quinidine gluconate. Usual doses of quinidine sulfate are 200 to 300 mg given orally three to four times a day (123,124). Before one interprets quinidine plasma concentrations, it is essential to determine the specificity of the assay used by the clinical laboratory; to evaluate the patient's clinical response to quinidine; and to assess the patient for the presence of congestive heart failure, liver disease, nephrotic syndrome or recent stress, all of which may alter the protein binding and clearance of this drug.

Therapeutic Plasma Concentrations

A number of quinidine assays of varying specificity are available. Each is associated with a different therapeutic range. Patients with quinidine levels higher than the upper limit of the therapeutic range are at greater risk for toxicity.

Protein Precipitation Assay. This is one of the oldest of the quinidine assays. It measures the fluorescence of a protein-free plasma filtrate and is nonspecific, measuring many less active metabolites in addition to quinidine (118,119). Assay concentrations of 4 to 8 mcg/ml correlate with therapeutic response (117).

Benzene Double Extraction Assay. This assay eliminates many but not all of the metabolites measured by the protein precipitation assay (26,118,120). Assay concentrations of 2 to 5 mcg/ml are therapeutic (35).

Specific Assays. These usually measure quinidine by high performance liquid chromatography (10,121), thin layer chromatography coupled with a fluorometric procedure (155) or enzyme

---

KEY PARAMETERS

Therapeutic Plasma Concentrations
  Specific Assays: 1–4 mcg/ml
  Benzene Double Extraction Assay: 2–5 mcg/ml
  Protein Precipitation Assay: 4–8 mcg/ml

	Vd (specific assays*)	Cl (specific assays*)	$t\frac{1}{2}$ (specific assays*)
Normal	2.7–3.0 L/kg	4.7 ml/min/kg (20 L/hr/70 kg)	7hrs
Congestive Heart Failure	1.8 L/kg	3.0–3.9 ml/min/kg (12–16 L/hr/70 kg)	7 hrs
Chronic Liver Disease	3.8 L/kg	decreased	increased
Nephrotic Patients	increased	increased	7 hrs

	S	F
Quinidine Sulfate	0.82	0.73
Quinidine Gluconate	0.62	0.70
Quinidine Polygalacturonate	0.62	?

---

*Since the benzene extraction and protein precipitation assays report higher plasma concentrations of quinidine, the calculated values for Vd and Cl will both be reduced. The decrease in these calculated parameters can be seen from the relationship between plasma concentration and volume of distribution:

$$Vd = \frac{Ab \text{ (or dose)}}{Cp} \qquad \text{(Eq. 9)}$$

and the relationship between plasma concentration and clearance:

$$Cl = \frac{(S)(F)(Dose/\tau)}{Cpss \text{ ave}} \qquad \text{(Eq. 14)}$$

Furthermore, "quinidine" levels measured by the protein precipitation assay include both quinidine and its metabolites and this may result in pharmacokinetic calculations that are misleading. For example, with only about 20% of quinidine cleared by the renal route (156), renal failure would not be expected to significantly prolong the half-life; yet, the accumulation of metabolites in renal failure has resulted in spuriously long estimates of quinidine half-life in patients with renal failure when the protein precipitate assay was used. This does not occur when the benzene double extraction assay is used (35).

immunoassay. Concentrations of 1 to 4 mcg/ml are therapeutic for these assays (10).

Changes in **plasma protein binding** due to chronic liver or kidney disease can also alter the desired therapeutic concentrations of quinidine. Quinidine is a basic drug which is bound primarily to alpha-1-acid glycoprotein (8). Although earlier studies suggested that quinidine was 80 to 90% bound to plasma proteins (alpha or fraction free = 0.2 to 0.1) (8,125), more recent studies indicate that the alpha or fraction free is approximately 0.1 for most patients (126). Since only the free or unbound drug is active, a change in the plasma protein binding could change the desired plasma concentration (see Part One, section on Desired Plasma Concentrations).

The plasma protein binding of quinidine is reduced in patients with *chronic liver disease,* presumably because of decreased alpha-1-acid glycoprotein concentration (121,127). Therefore the alpha or fraction free is increased and the desired quinidine plasma concentrations for patients with chronic liver disease will be lower than usual. (See Part One, Fig. 4).

The situation for *nephrotic patients* should be similar, although this group has not been studied. Nephrotic patients frequently have decreased alpha-1-acid glycoprotein concentrations in addition to hypoalbuminemia (128). Although a decrease in plasma proteins will decrease the desired therapeutic concentrations, the dosage regimen would remain the same (see Part One, Fig. 4).

The plasma protein binding of quinidine is increased following *acute stress* such as surgery (8). Such an event would tend to increase the total drug concentration with relatively little change in the free drug levels. For this reason, it would not be unusual to observe a normal therapeutic response in association with an elevated quinidine concentration in such patients.

Bioavailability

The bioavailability of quinidine is about 73% (F = 0.73) (155), but a range of 47% to 96% has been reported (121,155). Because quinidine is rapidly absorbed and has a short half-life which requires frequent dosing, some clinicians prefer to use sustained release preparations. These preparations also reduce the frequency of gastrointestinal side effects; however, the bioavailability of quinidine from these preparations may be lower than that of the non-sustained release products.

Volume of Distribution

The apparent volume of distribution of quinidine is 2.7 to 3.0 L/kg (121,122,156). There is an initial volume of distribution of 1.0 L/kg (156) but the distribution half-life is so brief (6 to 12 minutes) that this initial volume is of no consequence following oral administration (121,122,156).

In patients with *congestive heart failure,* the volume of distribution of quinidine is decreased to about 1.8 L/kg (121,122). The plasma protein binding of quinidine is decreased in patients with *chronic liver disease* and therefore the volume of distribution is increased (see Part One, Fig. 6 and section on Volume Distribution). The average volume of distribution of quinidine in patients with chronic liver disease is about 3.8 L/kg (127) although a volume of distribution as large as 9.7 L/kg has been observed in one patient (121). Since decreased plasma protein binding also occurs in *nephrotic patients* (128), they too would be expected to have larger volumes of distribution for quinidine.

Clearance

The average clearance for quinidine is about 4.7 ml/min/kg or about 20 L/hr/70 kg (121,156). Most of this is due to metabolism; only about 20% is cleared renally (121,156).

Quinidine clearance is decreased in *congestive heart failure,* presumably because of diminished hepatic blood flow. Quinidine clearance in patients with congestive heart failure is 3.0 to 3.9 ml/min/kg or 12 to 16 L/hr/70 kg (121,122).

Quinidine clearance is also decreased in *liver disease.* Clearance values calculated from total plasma quinidine concentrations in patients with chronic liver disease may look normal, but calculations which are based on the increased free drug concentration in these patients reveal impaired metabolic capacity (121,127). (Part One, section on Clearance: Plasma Protein Binding).

Elimination Half-Life

The usual half-life of quinidine is about 7 hours (121,156). The half-life is not affected by *congestive heart failure* because the volume of distribution and clearance are decreased by about the same proportion:

$$t\frac{1}{2} = \frac{(0.693)(\downarrow Vd)}{\downarrow Cl} \qquad \text{(Eq. 28)}$$

The half-life is increased in *chronic liver disease* because of a diminished metabolic capacity and increased volume of distribution:

$$t\frac{1}{2} = \frac{(0.693)(\uparrow Vd)}{\downarrow Cl} \qquad \text{(Eq. 28)}$$

In *renal failure*, the accumulation of metabolites which are reported as quinidine by the protein precipitation assay may erroneously suggest a significantly prolonged half-life (35).

1. R.M. is a 70 kg male with congestive heart failure and atrial fibrillation. He is to be given quinidine sulfate 300 mg orally every six hours. When should a plasma sample for quinidine concentration be obtained?

Since the half-life of quinidine is approximately seven hours and four half-lives are required to reach 93.75% of steady state, the plasma concentration should be evaluated after about 28 hours. As with most other drugs, the best time to evaluate plasma levels is just prior to a dose. This avoids many of the potential problems associated with delayed absorption and the uncertainty of when a peak concentration will occur following an oral dose (Part One, section on Interpretation of Plasma Drug Concentrations).

2. What plasma concentration would be expected in R.M. if a specific assay for quinidine is used? Is the prescribed regimen likely to maintain his quinidine levels within the therapeutic range?

Since the plasma sample will be obtained immediately prior to a dose, the reported level will be a trough or minimum level which can be predicted using Eq. 39:

$$\text{Cpss min} = \frac{\dfrac{(S)(F)(Dose)}{Vd}}{(1 - e^{-Kd\tau})} \times (e^{-Kd\tau}) \qquad \text{(Eq. 39)}$$

In this case S will be 0.82 since only 82% of quinidine sulfate is quinidine base. The following pharmacokinetic parameters can be used for R.M. who has congestive heart failure: F = 0.73 (156), Cl = 3 ml/min/kg (122) or 12.6 L/hr, Vd = 1.8 L/kg (122) or 126 L, Dose = 300 mg, and τ = 6 hr. Kd can be determined from Equation 23:

$$Kd = \frac{Cl}{Vd} \qquad \text{(Eq. 23)}$$

$$= \frac{12.6 \text{ L/hr}}{126 \text{ L}}$$

$$= 0.1 \text{ hr}^{-1}$$

Assuming these values are correct for R.M., the predicted level would be:

$$\text{Cpss min} = \frac{\dfrac{(S)(F)(Dose)}{Vd}}{(1 - e^{-Kd\tau})} \times (e^{-Kd\tau}) \qquad \text{(Eq. 39)}$$

$$= \frac{\dfrac{(0.73)(0.82)(300 \text{ mg})}{126 \text{ L}}}{1 - e^{-(0.1)(6)}} \times e^{-(0.1)(6)}$$

$$= \frac{1.43 \text{ mg/L}}{1 - e^{-0.6}} \times e^{-0.6}$$

$$= \frac{1.43 \text{ mg/L}}{1 - 0.55} \times 0.55$$

$$= \frac{1.43 \text{ mg/L}}{0.45} \times 0.55$$

$$= 1.75 \text{ mg/L (mcg/ml)}$$

This is within the therapeutic range of 1 to 4 mcg/ml. An estimation of the peak plasma concentration can also be made to insure that it will not be greater than the upper limit of the therapeutic range:

$$\text{Cpss max} = \frac{\dfrac{(S)(F)(Dose)}{Vd}}{(1 - e^{-Kd\tau})} \qquad \text{(Eq. 36)}$$

$$= \frac{\dfrac{(0.73)(0.82)(300 \text{ mg})}{126 \text{ L}}}{1 - e^{-(0.1)(6)}}$$

$$= \frac{1.43 \text{ mg/L}}{1 - e^{-0.6}}$$

$$= \frac{1.43 \text{ mg/L}}{1 - 0.55}$$

$$= 3.18 \text{ mg/L (mcg/ml)}$$

On the basis of these calculations it would be predicted that the prescribed regimen will produce plasma concentrations that are within the therapeutic range. Since these calculations were based upon the assumption that the drug was administered as intermittent intravenous boluses, oral administration should result in peak levels which are slightly lower and trough levels which are slightly higher than predicted. See Part One, Fig. 19.

3. The trough quinidine level reported for R.M. 28 hours after the regimen was initiated was 1.5 mcg/ml. Although this level is close to the predicted value and within the therapeutic range, R.M. did not have a satisfactory therapeutic response. The dose was increased from 300 to 400 mg every six hours and a second trough level obtained 15 days later was reported as 3.0 mcg/ml. Discounting error in the sampling time and the assay, what are possible explanations for the disproportionate rise in the plasma level?

The assumed volume of distribution and clearance may have been in error and the true half-life of quinidine in R.M. may be longer than the expected 7 hours. Since the quinidine level was obtained approximately 28 hours after starting the first regimen, the observed level of 1.5 mcg/ml may not have represented steady state. There is also the possibility that his clinical status has changed. Perhaps his heart failure worsened and decreased his quinidine clearance. Or, he may have had an injury or surgery that increased his alpha-1-acid glycoprotein concentration and thereby increased his plasma protein binding of quinidine (8).

In addition, there are recent reports of quinidine displaying dose-dependent or capacity-limited metabolism. Bolme and Otto noted that when quinidine sulfate doses were increased 50%, from 600 to 900 mg per day, the steady state quinidine concentration rose 94%. Furthermore, when the dose was increased another 33%, from 900 to 1200 mg per day, the steady state plasma concentrations rose 55% (129).

4. What dosage adjustment is required for patients receiving hemodialysis?

Since quinidine is highly bound to plasma protein and has a relatively large volume of distribution, significant removal would not be expected during dialysis. Two studies have verified this, demonstrating that no dosage adjustment is required for patients with end stage renal failure receiving hemodialysis (35,121). However, removal of the more polar metabolites by dialysis would be expected to result in a decrease in the plasma concentrations reported by nonspecific assays (121).

5. S.F., a 52-year-old male with a long history of alcohol abuse and cirrhosis developed premature ventricular contractions and heart failure. He is to be given quinidine. Establish a reasonable starting dose and target quinidine concentration for S.F.

This patient is complex because he has both congestive heart failure and liver disease. Patients with chronic liver disease have been reported to have an increased free fraction of quinidine because their concentrations of alpha-1-acid glycoprotein are low (see Part One, Fig. 4). In fact, the free fraction or alpha may be increased by as much as two or three times. Therefore, if the same free or unbound concentration of quinidine is desired, the therapeutic range should be reduced to one-half or one-third the usual value of 1 to 4 mcg/ml (121,127). As a first estimate, it would not be unreasonable to halve the usual maintenance dose of 200 mg every 6 hours and calculate the maximum and minimum plasma concentrations which would be produced by this reduced dosage regimen (100 mg every 6 hours).

However, it should be kept in mind that the pharmacokinetic parameters used to calculate the concentrations which will be produced by this regimen must also be adjusted for the patient's congestive heart failure and liver disease. The volume of distribution will be decreased by the congestive heart failure and increased by the low protein concentration in proportion to the change in alpha (see Part One, Fig. 6) (121). Clearance would be increased by the decreased protein binding (see Part One, Figs. 11 and 12), but reduced by both congestive heart failure and chronic liver disease (121).

The degree to which the clearance and volume of distribution should be adjusted in this patient is speculative, but doubling the volume of distribution observed in patients with congestive heart failure (2 × 1.8 L/kg) and leaving the clearance unchanged (since it is increased by the increase in alpha and decreased by liver disease and congestive heart failure), would not be unreasonable.

Using a volume of distribution of 3.6 L/kg and a clearance of 14 L/hr, the steady state peak and trough concentrations which would be produced by a dose of 100 mg of quinidine sulfate every 6 hours can be calculated:

$$Kd = \frac{Cl}{Vd} \qquad \text{(Eq. 23)}$$

$$= \frac{14 \text{ L/hr}}{(3.6 \text{ L/kg})(60 \text{ kg})}$$

$$= 0.065 \text{ hr}^{-1}$$

$$Cpss \text{ max} = \frac{(S)(F)(Dose)/Vd}{1 - e^{-Kd\tau}} \qquad \text{(Eq. 36)}$$

$$= \frac{(0.82)(0.72)(100 \text{ mg})/216 \text{ L}}{1 - e^{-(0.056/hr)(6 \text{ hr})}}$$

$$= 0.85 \text{ mg/L or } 0.85 \text{ mcg/ml}$$

$$\text{Cpss min} = (\text{Cpss max})(e^{-K_d\tau}) \qquad \qquad \text{(Eq. 38)}$$

$$= 0.85 \text{ mg/L} \times e^{-(0.056/hr)(6 \text{ hr})}$$

$$= 0.58 \text{ mg/L or } 0.58 \text{ mcg/ml}$$

Although the predicted peak and trough levels of 0.85 mcg/ml and 0.58 mcg/ml are below the usual therapeutic range of 1 to 4 mcg/ml, the decreased plasma protein binding (increased alpha) should produce free or unbound quinidine concentrations which are therapeutic. That is, if it is assumed that alpha increased two-fold in this patient, equivalent quinidine concentrations in the presence of normal protein levels would be twice as high as those calculated (Cpss max = 1.7 mcg/ml and Cpss min = 1.16 mcg/ml). These would be within the therapeutic range of 1 to 4 mcg. If it is subsequently found that the measured concentrations of quinidine are significantly greater than the predicted values, the intrinsic metabolic capability of the liver may be even worse than assumed or the plasma protein may be closer to normal than assumed. Since the degree to which quinidine binds to plasma protein is seldom known and it is difficult to quantitate liver function, the clinical status of the patient must be carefully evaluated before a change in the quinidine dosing regimen is considered.

6. P.C. is receiving 200 mg of quinidine sulfate orally every six hours. Calculate an equivalent intramuscular dose of quinidine gluconate.

To determine a dose of intramuscular quinidine gluconate which is equivalent to quinidine sulfate, the salt form (S) and bioavailability (F) of both dosage forms must be considered. Quinidine sulfate is 82% quinidine base (S = 0.82) and has a bioavailability of 73% (F = 0.73), while quinidine gluconate is 62% quinidine base (S = 0.62) and is probably completely absorbed (F = 1.0) when given parenterally. Eq. 3 can be used to calculate the amount of quinidine reaching the systemic circulation following the administration of an oral quinidine sulfate dose.

Amount of Drug Absorbed
or Reaching the Systemic $= (S)(F)(Dose)$ (Eq. 3)
Circulation

$$= (0.82)(0.73)(200 \text{ mg})$$

$$= 119.7 \text{ mg}$$

Eq. 2 can be modified by including the salt form (S) in the denominator so that the equivalent dose of intramuscular quinidine gluconate can be calculated:

$$\frac{\text{Dose of New}}{\text{Dosage Form}} = \frac{\begin{array}{c}\text{Amount of Drug Absorbed from}\\ \text{Current Dosage Form}\end{array}}{(S)(F) \text{ of New Dosage Form}} \quad \text{(Eq. 2)}$$

$$= \frac{119.7 \text{ mg}}{(0.62)(1)}$$

$$= 193 \text{ mg or approximately 200 mg}$$

As can be seen, the oral dose of quinidine sulfate and the intramuscular dose of quinidine gluconate are similar due to the offsetting effects of their bioavailabilities and salt forms.

6

Theophylline

Because of its ability to relax the smooth muscles of the bronchi, theophylline is widely used in the treatment of bronchial asthma and other respiratory diseases. The water solubility of theophylline is only about 1%; therefore it can be given parenterally only as aminophylline, the ethylenediamine salt of theophylline. There are a number of oral preparations of theophylline, aminophylline, and other theophylline salts. Aminophylline and other theophylline salts are sometimes administered rectally as suppositories or rectal solutions. Although still slow and erratic, the rectal solutions tend to have better absorption characteristics than do the suppositories.

Dosages vary widely and should be based upon pharmacokinetic considerations and plasma theophylline concentration determinations. Aminophylline is the most widely used salt of theophylline. In treating an average 70 kg patient with intractable bronchial asthma, a loading dose in the range of 250 to 500 mg is given by slow intravenous injection. This is followed by an intravenous aminophylline infusion given at a rate of about 30 to 50 mg per hour. Oral maintenance with aminophylline tablets is often in the range of 200 to 300 mg four times a day.

Therapeutic and Toxic Plasma Concentrations

The usually accepted therapeutic range for theophylline is 10 to 20 mcg/ml (mg/L) (38,159,160). However, improvement in respiratory function can be observed with plasma concentrations as low as 5 mcg/ml (38).

The most commonly observed side effects from theophylline are nausea and vomiting. Although nausea and vomiting occur at concentrations as low as 13 to 15 mcg/ml, they are much more frequent when the theophylline plasma concentration exceeds 20

KEY PARAMETERS	
Therapeutic Concentrations	10–20 mcg/ml
F[a]	100%
Vd[b]	0.48 L/kg
Cl[b]	0.04 L/hr/kg
t½	8.3 hr

[a] See Table 1
[b] Total body weight should be used for obese patients. (This recommendation differs from that of reference 229 which suggests that ideal body weight be used to estimate Vd.)
[c] See Table 2

mcg/ml (12,160). Cardiac symptoms such as tachycardia and premature atrial and ventricular contractions are less predictable but are usually associated with theophylline levels greater than 40 mcg/ml (161). Insomnia and nervousness are individual side effects which occur over a wide range of concentrations. Seizures are more severe CNS manifestations which usually occur at plasma concentrations exceeding 50 mcg/ml (161,162), although they have been observed in patients with theophylline concentrations below 30 mcg/ml (162,163).

Side effects such as nausea and vomiting which usually occur at lower plasma concentrations cannot be used as a reliable indication that excessive theophylline concentrations have been achieved. Furthermore, less severe toxic effects do not always occur at high concentrations. In a series of eight patients with theophylline-induced seizures, only one patient had premonitory signs and symptoms such as nausea, vomiting, tachycardia, or nervousness prior to the seizure (162).

Bioavailability

The bioavailability of the various dosage forms of theophylline is summarized in Table 1.

Volume of Distribution

The usual volume of distribution of theophylline is approximately 0.4 to 0.5 L/kg (4,161,164). Distribution follows a two-

Table 1
THEOPHYLLINE DOSAGE FORMS AND THEIR BIOAVAILABILITY

Dosage Form	S	F
Uncoated tablets and liquid		
Aminophylline	0.8 to 0.84	1.0
Elixophylline®	1.0	1.0
Theophylline	1.0	1.0
Coated and sustained release		
Choledyl® 100	0.64	1.0
200	0.64	0.9
Aminodur®	0.84	0.65
Aerolate®	1.0	0.81
Slophyllin Gyrocap®	1.0	1.0
Theobid Dura Cap®	1.0	0.87
Theodur®	1.0	1.0
Theophyl-SR®	1.0	1.0

S = Fraction of labeled dose which is theophylline
F = Fraction of theophylline absorbed
Adapted in part from Weinberger et al (3)

compartment model (see Part One, section on Volume of Distribution). The bronchioles behave as though they are located in the second or tissue compartment; however, toxicities may be related to high concentrations in the initial volume of distribution and may occur as a result of rapid administration and accumulation in that compartment.

Clearance

The average theophylline clearance is 0.04 L/hr/kg, based on lean or ideal body weight (4). A number of factors will influence theophylline clearance. The most common ones are summarized in Table 2.

Smokers have a theophylline clearance which is about 1.5 to 2 times as large as that of non-smokers (4,18,166). The effects of smoking (one pack of cigarettes per day) appear to last several months after the cigarettes have been discontinued. (166). Therefore, patients admitted to the hospital with a history of smoking should be considered as smokers throughout their hospitalization even if they refrain from smoking during that time.

Table 2
DISEASE STATES WHICH AFFECT THEOPHYLLINE CLEARANCE

Disease	Factor*	References
Smoking history	1.6	4, 166
Congestive heart failure	0.4	4, 167, 168
Acute pulmonary edema	0.5	169
Hepatic cirrhosis	0.5	170
Severe obstructive pulmonary disease	0.8	4
Obesity	IBW**	165

* Indicates the estimate for clearance adjustments. The product of all the factors which are present should be multiplied by the average clearance value (0.04 L/hr/kg × wt in kg)
** IBW = ideal body weight should be used.

The presence of *congestive heart failure*, on the other hand, reduces theophylline clearance to about 40% (4,167,168). Pulmonary edema has also been reported to cause a reduction in theophylline clearance (169). This change in clearance may be secondary to the associated congestive heart failure. *Severe pulmonary disease* reduces theophylline clearance to about 85% of the average value (4). *Hepatic cirrhosis* has also been identified as a factor which can significantly reduce theophylline clearance (4,170). *Premature newborns* have a theophylline clearance that is very low even when adjusted for weight or surface area (21).

Drug Interactions. Macrolide antibiotics such as triacetyl-oleandomycin and erythromycin have been reported to reduce theophylline clearance by as much as 50% (171,172) although this interaction with erythromycin has been disputed (229). Phenobarbital increases theophylline metabolism in some individuals by about 30% (173), but this induction has not been observed by all investigators (174). Unfortunately, the predictability of clearance changes secondary to the addition of these drugs is poor, indicating that while some change may be expected, each patient will need to be evaluated individually. This concept applies to disease states as well.

1. A patient receiving an aminophylline infusion has a plasma theophylline concentration of 30 mcg/ml. If the ami-

nophylline infusion rate is decreased by one-half, so that the new plasma theophylline concentration is 15 mcg/ml, will the pharmacologic (bronchodilating) effect also be reduced by one-half?

No. The bronchodilating effect of theophylline is proportional to the log of the theophylline concentration (38). This means that in order to get a two-fold change in the bronchodilating effect, the theophylline concentration would have to be changed by ten-fold. A 50% reduction in the plasma theophylline concentration in this patient may be well tolerated since the bronchodilating effect will be decreased by much less than 50%. However, before any change in theophylline plasma concentration is considered, the clinical status of the patient must be assessed. In some cases a change may have serious consequences: toxicity may appear if an increase in plasma concentration is attempted or increased bronchospasm may occur if the concentration is reduced.

2. R.J., an 80 kg, 50-year-old male, is seen in the emergency room and is diagnosed as having asthma unresponsive to epinephrine. Estimate a loading dose of aminophylline which will produce a plasma theophylline concentration of 15 mcg/ml.

Assuming R.J. has received no recent aminophylline doses, Eq. 10 could be used to determine the loading dose:

$$\text{Loading Dose} = \frac{(Vd)(Cp)}{(S)(F)} \tag{Eq. 10}$$

The S for the salt form of aminophylline is either 0.80 or 0.84 depending on whether the hydrous (0.80) or anhydrous (0.84) form was used to compound the drug product. The usual volume of distribution for theophylline is approximately 0.4 to 0.5 L/kg (4,160,164). Assuming a volume of distribution of 0.48 L/kg (4), R.J.'s volume of distribution is 38.4 L:

$$(0.48 \text{ L/kg})(80 \text{ kg}) = 38.4 \text{ L}$$

and the calculated loading dose would be 720 mg:

$$\text{Loading Dose} = \frac{(Vd)(Cp)}{(S)(F)} \qquad \text{(Eq. 10)}$$

$$= \frac{(38.4 \text{ L})(15 \text{ mg/L})}{(0.8)(1.0)}$$

$$= \frac{576 \text{ mg}}{0.8}$$

$$= 720 \text{ mg}$$

This dose is somewhat larger than the usual 300 to 500 mg loading dose for two reasons. First, the target level of 15 mcg/ml (mg/L) is higher than the usual 10 mg/L (38) which can be achieved with a loading dose of 5 to 6 mg/kg of aminophylline. Second, the patient is larger than average and, therefore, should require a larger loading dose.

3. Would the calculation for the loading dose have been different if R.J. were obese, with an estimated ideal body weight of 60 kg?

No. Although the Food and Drug Administration recommends that ideal body weight be used to calculate the loading dose (50), it appears that the volume of distribution (major determinant of loading dose) correlates best with total body weight rather than with lean or ideal body weight. While the average volume of distribution among obese patients is slightly smaller than that of non-obese patients, this difference was not considered to be significant by the investigators (165).

4. What factors will influence the theophylline loading dose?

The only factor which is known to influence the loading dose of theophylline is the presence of an initial plasma theophylline concentration. The presence of an initial plasma theophylline concentration can be accounted for in the calculation of a loading dose by using Eq. 11:

$$\text{Loading Dose} = \frac{(Vd)(Cp \text{ desired} - Cp \text{ initial})}{(S)(F)} \qquad \text{(Eq. 11)}$$

The volume of distribution of theophylline is a reliable parameter that does not usually change significantly from patient to patient.

Since "stat" theophylline levels are not widely available, it is common clinical practice to obtain a plasma sample and to administer approximately 3 mg/kg of aminophylline as a loading dose if the patient gives a history of having taken aminophylline within the past 12 to 24 hours. This reduced loading dose increases the plasma theophylline concentration by about 5 mg/L (mcg/ml), results in some bronchodilating effect even if the initial plasma theophylline concentration is zero and, hopefully, will not cause toxicity if the patient's initial theophylline concentration is greater than 10 to 20 mg/L.

5. Assuming that the aminophylline loading dose is to be given intravenously, how rapidly should it be administered?

Theophylline displays two-compartment pharmacokinetics in which the therapeutic or bronchodilating effects correlate more closely with concentrations in the second or tissue compartment (92). However, since toxic effects correlate with high concentrations in the initial volume of distribution, the loading dose should be infused over 30 minutes to minimize accumulation within this compartment and to avoid toxicity (37,38,164).

6. R.J., the 80 kg 50-year-old patient described in Question 2, received the 720 mg loading dose of aminophylline, and a theophylline plasma concentration of 15 mcg/ml (mg/L) was achieved. Estimate an aminophylline infusion rate which will maintain an average steady state level of 15 mcg/ml.

Since this problem involves a constant infusion which will be given to maintain a steady state plasma concentration, Eq. 15 can be used:

$$\text{Maintenance Dose} = \frac{(Cl)(Cpss\ ave)(\tau)}{(S)(F)} \qquad \text{(Eq. 15)}$$

Using an average theophylline clearance of 0.04 L/hr/kg (4), R.J.'s theophylline clearance would be 3.2 L/hr:

$$(0.04 \text{ L/hr/kg})(80 \text{ kg}) = 3.2 \text{ L/hr}$$

Again assuming aminophylline to be 80% theophylline (S = 0.80) and the bioavailability to be 100% (F = 1.0), the maintenance dose would be 60 mg/hr of aminophylline:

$$\text{Maintenance Dose} = \frac{(Cl)(Cpss\ ave)(\tau)}{(S)(F)} \qquad \text{(Eq. 15)}$$

$$= \frac{(3.2 \text{ L/hr})(15 \text{ mg/L})(1 \text{ hr})}{(0.8)(1.0)}$$

$$= \frac{48 \text{ mg}}{0.8}$$

$$= 60 \text{ mg aminophylline}$$

7. Would the calculated maintenance dose have been different if R.J. had been obese and his ideal body weight was 60 kg?

Unlike the volume of distribution, the clearance of theophylline seems to correlate better with ideal body weight than with total body weight (165). If R.J.'s ideal body weight was 60 kg, the clearance would be assumed to be 2.4 L/hr:

$$(0.04 \text{ L/hr/kg})(60 \text{ kg}) = 2.4 \text{ L/hr}$$

and the maintenance dose would therefore have been calculated to be 45 mg/hr of aminophylline:

$$\text{Maintenance Dose} = \frac{(Cl)(Cpss\ ave)(\tau)}{(S)(F)} \qquad \text{(Eq. 15)}$$

$$= \frac{(2.4 \text{ L/hr})(15 \text{ mg/L})(1 \text{ hr})}{(0.8)(1.0)}$$

$$= \frac{36 \text{ mg}}{0.8}$$

$$= 45 \text{ mg aminophylline}$$

8. **Assume that R.J. (80 kg ideal body weight) has a history of smoking more than a pack of cigarettes per day and also has severe obstructive pulmonary disease and congestive heart failure. Calculate a maintenance dose of aminophylline which will maintain the average steady state theophylline plasma concentration at 15 mcg/ml (mg/L).**

If none of the factors listed in Table 2 were present, R.J.'s expected theophylline clearance would be 3.2 L/hr:

$$(0.04 \text{ L/hr/kg})(80 \text{ kg}) = 3.2 \text{ L/hr}$$

Referring to Table 2, the factors present in R.J. which alter clearance include smoking, severe obstructive pulmonary disease and congestive heart failure. These alter clearance by a factor of 1.6, 0.4, and 0.8 respectively. The product of these factors is 0.512:

$$(1.6)(0.4)(0.8) = 0.512$$

This factor of 0.512 should then be multiplied by the average theophylline clearance value to estimate the theophylline clearance for this patient:

$$(3.2 \text{ L/hr})(0.512) = 1.64 \text{ L/hr}$$

This clearance could then be used in Eq. 15 to calculate the maintenance dose:

$$\text{Maintenance Dose} = \frac{(Cl)(Cpss \text{ ave})(\tau)}{(S)(F)} \qquad \text{(Eq. 15)}$$

$$= \frac{(1.64 \text{ L/hr})(15 \text{ mg/L})(1 \text{ hr})}{(0.8)(1.0)}$$

$$= \frac{24.6 \text{ mg}}{0.8}$$

$$= 30.75 \text{ mg}$$

Therefore, the estimated maintenance dose for this patient would be about 30 mg of aminophylline every hour.

9. Approximate R.J.'s theophylline half-life, assuming the clearance is 1.64 L/hr (as calculated in Question 8) and the volume of distribution is 38.4 L (as calculated in Question 2).

The half-life is a function of clearance and volume of distribution and can be calculated using Eq. 28:

$$t\frac{1}{2} = \frac{(0.693)(Vd)}{Cl}$$ (Eq. 28)

$$= \frac{(0.693)(38.4 \text{ L})}{1.64 \text{ L/hr}}$$

$$= \frac{26.6 \text{ L}}{1.64 \text{ L/hr}}$$

$$= 16.2 \text{ hours}$$

This half-life is considerably longer than the average of 6 to 10 hours because of the disease states present.

10. At what point after starting the infusion should a theophylline plasma concentration be obtained?

Even though the expected theophylline half-life for this patient is 16 hours, the optimal time to obtain a plasma sample for theophylline concentration would still be 12 to 20 hours after starting the maintenance infusion (approximately 2 times the usual half-life). The object of taking a sample early is to minimize the time during which low plasma concentrations will exist if the clearance is greater than expected and to prevent excessive accumulation if the clearance is less than expected.

However, plasma theophylline concentrations obtained within one half-life cannot be reliably used to calculate clearance or Cpss ave since both of these values are very sensitive to small errors in the assay and estimates of the volume of distribution when they are derived from such samples. If the theophylline concentration at 12 to 20 hours is significantly higher than expected (clearance is less than expected), the infusion rate should be reduced at that time. A second plasma concentration should then be obtained the following day to re-evaluate the patient's clearance and predicted steady state concentration.

11. M.K., a 58-year-old 63 kg woman, was admitted to the hospital in status asthmaticus. She received an intravenous aminophylline loading dose of 375 mg at 9 pm, followed by a constant aminophylline infusion of 60 mg/hr. The next morning at 7 am (10 hours after the bolus and initiation of the infusion) a plasma sample was obtained and the reported theophylline concentration was 18 mcg/ml. Calculate the apparent clearance and half-life of theophylline in this patient.

It is unlikely that the reported plasma concentration of 18 mcg/ml represents a steady state concentration, since the sample was obtained only 10 hours after the infusion was begun. The plasma concentration versus time curve which describes a bolus followed by a constant infusion and the plasma concentration which is produced by this mode of administration is depicted in Part One, Fig. 24.

As illustrated in that figure, the reported plasma concentration of 18 mg/L is actually the sum of the plasma concentration produced by the loading dose and that produced by the infusion:

$$Cp_1 = \text{(loading dose and decay equation)} + \text{(infusion equation)}$$

$$18 \text{ mg/L} = \left[\frac{(S)(F)(Dose)}{Vd} \times e^{-Kdt_1} \right] + \left[\frac{(S)(F)(Dose/\tau)}{Cl} \times (1 - e^{-Kdt_1}) \right]$$

Assuming that S and F are 0.8 and 1.0 respectively, that t_1 is 10 hours, that the loading dose is 375 mg, Dose/τ is 60 mg/hr, Kd = Cl/Vd (see Eq. 23), and that Vd = 0.48 L/kg or 30L for this 63 kg patient, the above equation can be reduced to:

$$18 \text{ mg/L} = \left[\frac{(0.8)(1.0)(375 \text{ mg})}{Vd} \times e^{-\left(\frac{Cl}{Vd}\right)(10 \text{ hr})} \right] + \left[\frac{(0.8)(1.0)(60 \text{ mg/hr})}{Cl} \times 1 - e^{-\left(\frac{Cl}{Vd}\right)(10 \text{ hr})} \right]$$

$$= \left[10 \text{ mg/L} \times e^{-\left(\frac{Cl}{30 \text{ L}}\right)(10 \text{ hr})} \right] + \left[\frac{48 \text{ mg/hr}}{Cl} + 1 - e^{-\left(\frac{Cl}{30 \text{ L}}\right)(10 \text{ hr})} \right]$$

Unfortunately, clearance cannot be solved for directly, but must be determined through trial and error by finding a value which will result in a theophylline concentration of 18 mg/L. If one has a good clinical history, the factors in Table 2 should aid in making the initial estimate for clearance. In this case no history is provided, so a clearance of 0.04 L/hr/kg could be tried in the above equation. However, application of this clearance to Eq. 31 would result in a final steady state theophylline concentration of only 19 mcg/ml:

$$(0.04 \text{ L/hr/kg})(63 \text{ kg}) = 2.52 \text{ L/hr}$$

$$\text{Cpss ave} = \frac{(S)(F)(\text{Dose}/\tau)}{Cl} \qquad \text{(Eq. 31)}$$

$$= \frac{(0.8)(1.0)(60 \text{ mg/1 hr})}{2.52 \text{ L/hr}}$$

$$= 19 \text{ mg/L}$$

It is unlikely that a theophylline concentration which has increased from 10 to 18 mg/L (mcg/L) in 10 hours will plateau at 19 mg/L. Therefore the best clearance estimate is something less than 2.52 L/hr. Furthermore, if a clearance of 2.52 L/hr is inserted into the simplified equation, the predicted theophylline concentration at the 10 hours would only be 15 mg/L. Since the predicted theophylline concentration using a clearance of 2.52 L/hr is less than that which was observed, the patient's clearance must be less than this value. If a new clearance estimate of 2.0 L/hr is used, the calculated theophylline concentration at 10 hours is 17 mg/L:

$$Cp_{10 \text{ hr}} = \left[10 \text{ mg/L} \times e^{-(2.0/30)(10)} \right] + \left[\frac{48 \text{ mg/hr}}{2.0 \text{ L/hr}} \times 1 - e^{-(2.0/30)(10)} \right]$$

$$= \left[10 \text{ mg/L} \times e^{-0.66} \right] + \left[24 \text{ mg/L} \times 1 - e^{-0.66} \right]$$

$$= (10 \text{ mg/L})(0.51) + (24 \text{ mg/L})(1 - 0.51)$$

$$= 5.1 \text{ mg/L} + 11.8 \text{ mg/L}$$

$$= 16.9 \text{ mg/L or approximately 17 mg/L}$$

Since this predicted plasma theophylline concentration is also less than that which was observed, the clearance must be less than 2.0 L/hr. Further trials would demonstrate that a clearance value of 1.65 L/hr results in a predicted theophylline level of 18 mg/L.

Because the plasma theophylline sample was taken after about one usual theophylline half-life, the clearance estimate of 1.65 L/hr may contain some error. However, if it is assumed that this clearance estimate is correct, the calculated theophylline half-life would be 12.6 hours:

$$t\frac{1}{2} = \frac{(0.693)(Vd)}{Cl} \qquad \text{(Eq. 28)}$$

$$= \frac{(0.693)(30 \text{ L})}{1.65 \text{ L/hr}}$$

$$= 12.6 \text{ hours}$$

12. Assuming that the desired steady state plasma theophylline concentration for M.K. is less than 20 mcg/ml (mg/L), determine whether the maintenance dose needs to be adjusted.

Since clearance is the primary determinant of the steady state plasma concentration, this value can be used to estimate the plasma theophylline concentration which will be produced by an aminophylline infusion of 60 mg/hr:

$$Cpss \text{ ave} = \frac{(S)(F)(Dose/\tau)}{Cl} \qquad \text{(Eq. 31)}$$

$$= \frac{(0.8)(1.0)(60 \text{ mg/1 hr})}{1.65 \text{ L/hr}}$$

$$= \frac{48 \text{ mg/hr}}{1.65 \text{ L/hr}}$$

$$= 29 \text{ mg/L}$$

Since this predicted steady state plasma theophylline concentration of 29 mg/L exceeds 20 mg/L, the infusion rate should be adjusted. The new infusion rate can be calculated from Eq. 15 by inserting the desired steady state plasma concentration and using the clearance estimate of 1.65 L/hr. If a steady state plasma concentration of 15 mg/L is desired, the new maintenance infusion will be 30.9 mg/hr of aminophylline:

$$\text{Maintenance Dose} = \frac{(Cl)(Cpss\ ave)(\tau)}{(S)(F)} \qquad \text{(Eq. 15)}$$

$$= \frac{(1.65\ L/hr)(15\ mg/L)(1\ hr)}{(0.8)(1.0)}$$

$$= \frac{24.75\ mg}{0.8}$$

$$= 30.9\ mg/hr$$

In this case, it would be advisable to obtain another plasma theophylline concentration on the following morning after the infusion rate has been reduced to ensure that the clearance estimate of 1.65 L/hr is reasonably close to the actual value.

13. O.P., a 75 kg male patient, became nauseated after he had received an intravenous aminophylline infusion at a rate of 85 mg/hr for several days. A plasma sample for theophylline concentration was obtained and the infusion was discontinued. Twelve hours later a second plasma sample was obtained. The reported plasma theophylline concentrations were 32 and 16 mcg/ml (mg/L) respectively. Estimate the hourly dose of aminophylline required to maintain the plasma theophylline concentration at 15 mcg/ml (mg/L).

In this case there are two ways to calculate a new maintenance dose. One method would entail estimating the elimination rate constant from the decay pattern by use of Eq. 24 and to use this value and an assumed volume of distribution to calculate clearance, the major determinant of the maintenance dose. Once clearance is known, the new maintenance dose can be calculated using Eq. 15.

$$Kd = \frac{\ln\left(\dfrac{Cp_1}{Cp_2}\right)}{t} \qquad \text{(Eq. 24)}$$

where Cp_1 is 32 mg/L, Cp_2 is 16 mg/L and t is the 12 hours between the two plasma concentrations. Therefore,

$$Kd = \frac{\ln\left(\frac{32}{16}\right)}{12 \text{ hrs}}$$

$$= \frac{\ln(2)}{12 \text{ hrs}}$$

$$= \frac{0.693}{12 \text{ hrs}}$$

$$= 0.058 \text{ hrs}^{-1}$$

If the volume of distribution is assumed to be 0.48 L/kg or 36 L (0.48 L/kg × 75 kg = 36 L), the clearance can be estimated from Eq. 29:

$$Cl = (Kd)(Vd) \qquad \text{(Eq. 29)}$$

$$= (0.058 \text{ hrs}^{-1})(36 \text{ L})$$

$$= 2.1 \text{ L/hr}$$

Now, using Eq. 15, the maintenance dose can be calculated if it is assumed that S, F and τ are 0.8, 1.0 and 1 hr respectively:

$$\text{Maintenance Dose} = \frac{(Cl)(Cpss \text{ ave})(\tau)}{(S)(F)} \qquad \text{(Eq. 15)}$$

$$= \frac{(2.1 \text{ L/hr})(15 \text{ mg/L})(1 \text{ hr})}{(0.8)(1.0)}$$

$$= \frac{31.5 \text{ mg}}{0.8}$$

$$= 39.3 \text{ mg}$$

Thus, an aminophylline infusion of 40 mg per hour should result in a steady state plasma theophylline concentration of 15 mg/L.

A second and more direct method would have been to assume that the plasma concentration of 32 mg/L represented steady state and to calculate the apparent theophylline clearance directly by use of Eq. 14:

$$Cl = \frac{(S)(F)(Dose/\tau)}{Cpss\ ave} \qquad (Eq.\ 14)$$

$$= \frac{(0.8)(1.0)(85\ mg/1\ hr)}{32\ mg/L}$$

$$= \frac{68\ mg/hr}{32\ mg/L}$$

$$= 2.1\ L/hr$$

In this case both clearance estimates were the same. The first method should be used if steady state has not been achieved or if the dosing history is unreliable. However, this method requires a reasonable time interval (one half-life) between plasma samples so that the elimination rate constant can be calculated and a reliable estimate of the volume of distribution. The second method is preferred when the volume of distribution estimate is questionable or when an accurate estimate of the elimination rate constant cannot be made.

14. S.R. is a 70 kg, 40-year-old male who has been receiving an intravenous aminophylline infusion at a rate of 35 mg/hr. His steady state plasma theophylline concentration is 15 mg/L. Calculate an appropriate oral dosing regimen and estimate the peak and trough levels which would be produced by this regimen.

One method is to multiply the hourly intravenous dose by the dosing interval to be used for oral therapy. For example, if a six hour dosing interval is to be used for S.R., the equivalent oral dose would be 210 mg (35 mg/hr × 6 hrs = 210 mg) every six hours. It is assumed here that the same salt form (aminophylline) will be used and the bioavailability of the oral form is 100% (F = 1.0) (See Table 2). The usual aminophylline dosage form of 200 mg is reasonably close to the calculated dose of 210 mg and would probably be prescribed.

It is important to consider that the peak and trough plasma concentrations produced by intermittent dosing will be higher and lower than the average concentration achieved during the infusion. There are two methods of estimating Cpss max and Cpss min in this instance. *Method I:* A quick way to estimate the peak and trough plasma concentrations which will be produced when the *same average dose* is given on an intermittent schedule is to first calculate the expected difference between the peak and trough concentrations. Then, by adding half of this value to the average plasma concentration, the peak concentration can be estimated. Similarly, half of the difference between peak and trough concentrations can be subtracted from the average plasma concentration to estimate the trough concentration.

If aminophylline is administered at equal dosing intervals around the clock, all of a dose will be cleared prior to the administration of the next dose at steady state; that is, the rate in equals the rate out. Therefore each dose may be thought of as a loading dose that is repeated after the previous loading dose has been cleared from the body. The total plasma concentration after each dose is administered is the sum of the plasma concentration existing prior to the dose (trough concentration) and the increment in plasma concentration produced by that dose. If it is assumed that absorption is rapid the maximum difference between peak and trough plasma concentrations can be estimated by rearranging Eq. 10:

$$\text{Loading Dose} = \frac{(Vd)(Cp)}{(S)(F)} \qquad \text{(Eq. 10)}$$

$$Cp = \frac{(S)(F)(Dose)}{Vd}$$

In this case Cp is not the expected plasma concentration but the change or increment in plasma concentration produced by each dose (ΔCp). Assuming S is 0.8, F is 1.0, and Vd is 0.48 L/kg, each 200 mg dose of aminophylline should produce a 4.8 mg/L increment in the plasma theophylline concentration:

$$\Delta Cp = \frac{(S)(F)(Dose)}{Vd}$$

$$= \frac{(0.8)(1.0)(200 \text{ mg})}{(0.48 \text{ L/kg})(70 \text{ kg})}$$

$$= \frac{160 \text{ mg}}{33.6 \text{ L}}$$

$$= 4.8 \text{ mg/L}$$

One-half of this change in plasma concentration is 2.4 mg/L. Therefore the peak concentration produced by the prescribed regimen should be approximately 17.4 mg/L and the trough concentration should be 12.6 mg/L:

$$\text{Cpss max} = \text{Cpss ave} + \tfrac{1}{2}\Delta Cp$$
$$= 15 \text{ mg/L} + 2.4 \text{ mg/L}$$
$$= 17.4 \text{ mg/L}$$

$$\text{Cpss min} = \text{Cpss ave} - \tfrac{1}{2}\Delta Cp$$
$$= 15 \text{ mg/L} - 2.4 \text{ mg/L}$$
$$= 12.6 \text{ mg/L}$$

This approach assumes that the oral dose will produce the same average plasma concentration as the intravenous infusion, that the oral dosage form will be absorbed rapidly and completely and that the dosing interval is equal to or shorter than the theophylline half-life.

Method II: A second method which may be used to calculate the peak and trough plasma concentrations is to first estimate the clearance and volume of distribution and thereby the Kd in this patient and then to use Equations 36 and 38 to estimate the maximum and minimum plasma concentrations:

$$\text{Cpss max} = \frac{\dfrac{(S)(F)(Dose)}{Vd}}{(1 - e^{-Kd\tau})} \qquad \text{(Eq. 36)}$$

$$\text{Cpss min} = (\text{Cpss max})(e^{-Kd\tau}) \qquad \text{(Eq. 38)}$$

In order to use these equations, the Kd (elimination rate constant) must first be estimated. The theophylline Kd for S.R. is a function of his theophylline clearance and volume of distribution. The clearance can be calculated from the observed steady state plasma theophylline concentration:

$$Cl = \frac{(S)(F)(Dose/\tau)}{Cpss\ ave} \qquad \text{(Eq. 14)}$$

$$= \frac{(0.8)(1.0)(35\ mg/1\ hr)}{15\ mg/L}$$

$$= \frac{28\ mg/hr}{15\ mg/L}$$

$$= 1.87\ L/hr$$

Assuming the volume of distribution is 33.6 L (0.48 L/kg × 70 kg = 33.6L), the elimination rate constant can be calculated from Eq. 23:

$$Kd = \frac{Cl}{Vd} \qquad \text{(Eq. 23)}$$

$$= \frac{1.87\ L/hr}{33.6\ L}$$

$$= 0.056\ hr^{-1}$$

Based on this Kd of 0.056 hr^{-1}, a Vd of 33.6 L and a τ of 6 hrs, the calculated maximum plasma theophylline concentration after each 200 aminophylline dose is 16.79 mg/L:

$$Cpss\ max = \frac{\dfrac{(S)(F)(Dose)}{Vd}}{(1 - e^{-Kd\tau})} \qquad \text{(Eq. 36)}$$

$$= \frac{\dfrac{(0.8)(1.0)(200\ mg)}{33.6\ L}}{1 - e^{-(0.056\ hr^{-1})(6\ hr)}}$$

$$= \frac{\dfrac{160\ mg}{33.6\ L}}{1 - e^{-0.33}}$$

$$= \frac{4.76\ mg/L}{1 - 0.72}$$

$$= \frac{4.76\ mg/L}{0.28}$$

$$= 16.79\ mg/L$$

And the minimum plasma concentration prior to each dose would be 12.1 mg/L:

$$\text{Cpss min} = (\text{Cpss max})(e^{-K_d\tau}) \qquad \text{(Eq. 38)}$$

$$= [16.79 \text{ mg/L}][e^{-(0.056)(6)}]$$

$$= (16.79 \text{ mg/L})(e^{-0.33})$$

$$= (16.79 \text{ mg/L})(0.72)$$

$$= 12.1 \text{ mg/L}$$

These estimates are reasonably close to the previous estimates. They differ primarily because the average steady state theophylline concentration from the oral regimen will be slightly lower than the assumed 15 mg/L since the oral dose is 200 mg rather than the 210 mg (35 mg/hr × 6 hrs) which was given by intravenous infusion and because the average concentration is a little closer to the trough than the peak concentration.

15. What type of patients are likely to experience wide fluctuations in their plasma theophylline concentrations when taking oral doses every six hours?

Patients with a short theophylline half-life (i.e., less than six hours) will tend to have high peak plasma concentrations and low trough concentrations with a dosing interval of six hours or more. Since the volume of distribution of theophylline is reasonably constant, patients who clear theophylline at a high rate will have a short theophylline half-life:

$$t^{1/2} = \frac{(0.693)(\text{Vd})}{\text{Cl}} \qquad \text{(Eq. 28)}$$

In general, pediatric patients tend to have higher theophylline clearances and shorter theophylline half-lives than the average adult (175,176,177). Adults who smoke but do not have other complicating disease states such as congestive heart failure also tend to have theophylline half-lives which are shorter than six hours (18,166). To minimize wide fluctuations in the plasma theophylline concentration in these cases one should shorten the dosing interval or consider prescribing a sustained-release preparation.

16. When should plasma samples for theophylline concentrations be obtained for a patient who is on an oral regimen with a constant dosing interval?

Plasma samples should be obtained immediately prior to the scheduled dose because trough concentrations are more predictable than are peak concentrations. Peak plasma concentrations can be delayed by slow absorption, resulting in substantial error. See Part One, Fig. 20.

Since theophylline has a fairly short half-life in many patients, the difference between the trough and peak concentrations can be rather great. Therefore, a low trough concentration may be observed in patients with high peak concentrations. Also, toxicity is a frequent occurrence when the dose is increased to bring trough concentrations into the usually accepted therapeutic range of 10 to 20 mcg/ml. Such toxicity may be prevented by estimating the peak plasma concentration. This can be done by calculating the increment in plasma concentration which will be produced by each dose and adding it to the observed trough concentration. This principle is illustrated in the following question.

17. A patient who weighs 33 kg has been receiving 200 mg of aminophylline every six hours for several days. A plasma theophylline sample drawn immediately prior to a scheduled dose was reported as 5.0 mg/L. Estimate the peak plasma concentration after each dose.

The reported plasma theophylline concentration of 5.0 mg/L is a trough concentration. The peak plasma concentration will be the sum of this plasma concentration and the expected change in theophylline concentration resulting from each dose. The change in theophylline concentration can be calculated by rearranging Eq. 10 as was done in the first part of Question 4:

$$\text{Loading Dose} = \frac{(Vd)(Cp)}{(S)(F)} \qquad \text{(Eq. 10)}$$

$$Cp = \frac{(S)(F)(Dose)}{Vd}$$

Assuming the average Vd of 0.48 L/kg, the patient's Vd would be 15.84 L (0.48 L/kg × 33 kg = 15.84 L). Therefore,

$$Cp = \frac{(0.8)(1.0)(200 \text{ mg})}{15.84 \text{ L}}$$

$$= 10.1 \text{ mg/L}$$

Thus, each 200 mg dose of aminophylline will increase the trough theophylline concentration by approximately 10 mg/L, so the peak plasma concentration will be 15 mg/L (5 mg/L + 10 mg/L = 15 mg/L). Actually, the peak concentration will be somewhat lower than this since oral absorption will dampen the peak. It is important to note that if the dose is doubled to achieve a trough concentration of 10 mcg/ml, that the peak concentration would also be doubled to approximately 30 mcg/ml.

18. E.L. is a 50 kg patient receiving an aminophylline infusion of 50 mg/hr; his steady state plasma theophylline concentration is 15 mg/L. Parenteral aminophylline is being discontinued and oral aminophylline 300 mg on a 9 am, 1 pm, 5 pm, and 9 pm schedule has been prescribed. Do you anticipate any problems?

Because the average daily administration rate is the same (1200 mg/day) on both regimens, the *average* steady state level will be the same. However, because the interval between doses is irregular (every four hours between 9 am and 9 pm followed by an interval of twelve hours between 9 pm and 9 am), the plasma theophylline concentration will be increasing during the day and declining during the night and early morning hours (see Fig. 1).

The two plasma levels of most interest would be the peak concentration just after the 9 pm dose and the trough concentration just before the 9 am dose. These plasma levels should represent the highest and lowest levels achievable on this dosing regimen.

Since the dosing interval is irregular, the usual steady state Cpss max and Cpss min equations cannot be used. Instead, the plasma level at any given time may be thought of as the sum of that produced by four separate doses each of which is given every 24 hours (i.e., each 9 am dose is given every 24 hours, each 1 pm dose is given every 24 hours, etc.). The plasma level produced by any *one* of the four regimens at a given point in time is the Cpss max for that dose multiplied by the fraction of drug remaining at that point in time:

Cp = (Cpss max)(fraction remaining)

$$\text{Cpss max} = \frac{\dfrac{(S)(F)(Dose)}{Vd}}{1 - e^{-Kd\tau}} \qquad \text{(Eq. 36)}$$

$$\text{fraction remaining} = e^{-Kdt} \qquad \text{(Eq. 34)}$$

$$\text{therefore, Cp} = \frac{\dfrac{(S)(F)(Dose)}{Vd}}{1 - e^{-Kd\tau}} \times e^{-Kdt}$$

The actual plasma level at any given time is the *sum* of the levels produced by each of the four regimens. Since each regimen is given every 24 hours, τ is 24 hours.

$$Cp = \left[\frac{\dfrac{(S)(F)(Dose)}{Vd}}{1 - e^{-Kd(24\ hr)}} \right] [e^{-Kdt_1}] + \left[\frac{\dfrac{(S)(F)(Dose)}{Vd}}{1 - e^{-Kd(24\ hr)}} \right] [e^{-Kdt_2}] + \dots$$

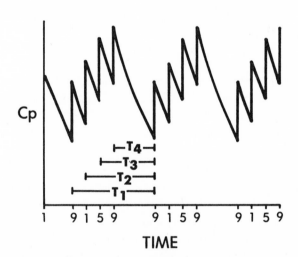

Fig. 1. Plasma level time curve for a dosing regimen of 9 AM, 1 PM, 5 PM and 9 PM. Note that plasma concentrations are lowest just prior to the 9 AM dose. In addition, even though the interval between doses is irregular, each dose is given every 24 hours, at 9 AM, 1 PM, 5 PM and 9 PM respectively.

Or, more simply stated:

$$Cp = \left[\frac{\frac{(S)(F)(Dose)}{Vd}}{1 - e^{-Kd(24\ hr)}} \right] [e^{-Kdt_1} + e^{-Kdt_2} + e^{-Kdt_3} + e^{-Kdt_4}]$$

where t_1, t_2, t_3, and t_4 represent the time intervals between the time of administration for each dose and the time at which one wishes to predict the plasma theophylline level.

To solve the above equation for Cp one must first calculate Kd which can be derived from the clearance and volume of distribution (see Eq. 23). Since a steady state level (15 mg/L) and dose (50 mg/hr) are known, clearance can be calculated through the use of Eq. 14:

$$Cl = \frac{(S)(F)(Dose/\tau)}{Cpss\ ave} \qquad \text{(Eq. 14)}$$

$$= \frac{(0.8)(1.0)(50\ mg/1\ hr)}{15\ mg/L}$$

$$= 2.67\ L/hr$$

If the volume of distribution is assumed to be 24 L (0.48 L/kg $\times$ 50 kg = 24 L), the elimination rate constant can be calculated as follows:

$$Kd = \frac{Cl}{Vd} \qquad \text{(Eq. 23)}$$

$$= \frac{2.67\ L/hr}{24\ L}$$

$$= 0.11\ hr^{-1}$$

The plasma level after the 9 pm dose can now be determined by considering t_1 through t_4 as the number of hours since the last 9 pm, 5 pm, 1 pm and 9 am doses were administered. Therefore, t_1 through t_4 would be 0, 4, 8, and 12 hours respectively, assuming the 9 pm dose had been administered and was rapidly absorbed.

$$\text{Cp at 9 pm} = \left[\frac{\dfrac{(0.8)(1.0)(300 \text{ mg})}{24 \text{ L}}}{1 - e^{-(0.11)(24)}} \right] \left[\begin{array}{l} [e^{-(0.11)(0 \text{ hr})} + e^{-(0.11)(4 \text{ hr})} \\ + e^{-(0.11)(8 \text{ hr})} + e^{-(0.11)(12 \text{ hr})}] \end{array} \right]$$

$$= \left[\frac{10 \text{ mg/L}}{1 - e^{-2.64}} \right] [e^{-0} + e^{-0.44} + e^{-0.88} + e^{-1.32}]$$

$$= \left[\frac{10 \text{ mg/L}}{1 - 0.071} \right] [1 + 0.64 + 0.41 + 0.27]$$

$$= \left[\frac{10 \text{ mg/L}}{0.929} \right] [2.32]$$

$$= 25 \text{ mg/L}$$

The level just before the 9 am dose could be calculated using the same equation and the appropriate time intervals. In this case the time intervals since the last 9 am, 1 pm, 5 pm and 9 pm dose would be 24 hours, 20 hours, 16 hours, and 12 hours respectively.

Another method which could be used to determine the level just prior to the morning dose would be to multiply the peak concentration of 25 mg/L by the fraction remaining after 12 hours:

$$\text{Cp} = (\text{Cp}^0)(e^{-Kdt}) \tag{Eq. 22}$$

$$\text{Cp} = (25 \text{ mg/L})(e^{-(0.11)(12)})$$

$$= (25 \text{ mg/L})(e^{-1.32})$$

$$= (25 \text{ mg/L})(0.27)$$

$$= 6.75 \text{ mg/L (immediately prior to 9 am dose)}$$

While it is possible that the patient could be well controlled clinically on this 9 am, 1 pm, 5 pm, 9 pm dosing schedule, a dosing interval of six hours would result in much lower peaks and higher trough concentrations, thus minimizing toxicity and maximizing therapeutic response:

$$\text{Cpss max} = \frac{\dfrac{(S)(F)(\text{Dose})}{Vd}}{(1 - e^{-Kd\tau})} \tag{Eq. 36}$$

$$= \frac{\dfrac{(0.8)(1.0)(300 \text{ mg})}{24 \text{ L}}}{1 - e^{-(0.11)(6 \text{ hr})}}$$

$$= \frac{10 \text{ mg/L}}{1 - e^{-0.66}}$$

$$= \frac{10 \text{ mg/L}}{1 - 0.52}$$

$$= \frac{10 \text{ mg/L}}{0.48}$$

$$= 20.8 \text{ mg/L}$$

$$\text{Cpss min} = (\text{Cpss max})(e^{-Kd\tau}) \qquad \text{(Eq. 37)}$$

$$= [20.8 \text{ mg/L}][e^{-(0.11)(6)}]$$

$$= (20.8 \text{ mg/L})(e^{-0.66})$$

$$= (20.8 \text{ mg/L})(0.52)$$

$$= 10.8 \text{ mg/L}$$

An alternative to the six hour dosing interval is the use of a sustained release product which can be administered less frequently. Such a product would minimize the fluctuation in theophylline plasma concentration between dosing intervals and would thus minimize the possibility of toxic peak levels and subtherapeutic trough levels in a patient who requires a high Cpss ave for clinical control.

19. If this patient were placed on a sustained release dosage form such as Theo-dur® 600 mg every 12 hours, how would you calculate the expected theophylline concentrations?

Assuming Theo-dur® has slow release characteristics, the plasma levels should not change very much even if the dosing interval is 12 hours. The administration of this oral form could thus be treated as an infusion and would therefore be described by Eq. 31.

$$\text{Cpss ave} = \frac{(S)(F)(\text{Dose}/\tau)}{Cl} \qquad \text{(Eq. 31)}$$

In this case S is 1.0 since Theo-dur® is labeled as containing theophylline rather than aminophylline and the F appears to be about 1.0 (3).

$$\text{Cpss ave} = \frac{(1.0)(1.0)(600 \text{ mg/12 hrs})}{2.67 \text{ L/hr}}$$

$$= \frac{50 \text{ mg/hr}}{2.67 \text{ L/hr}}$$

$$= 18.7 \text{ mg/L}$$

Calculation of peak and trough levels with Equations 36 and 38 would be inappropriate as the levels should fluctuate very little during the dosing interval.

7

Gentamicin

Gentamicin is a bactericidal antibiotic used in the treatment of serious gram-negative infections. Because it is poorly absorbed from the gastrointestinal tract, it is administered parenterally and occasionally topically. In most instances gentamicin is administered by intermittent intravenous infusion. Doses depend upon the etiologic agent, the renal function, and weight of the patient. Infusions of 100 mg given over a period of one hour and repeated every eight hours are not uncommon for a 70 kg individual.

The clearance, volume of distribution and half-life of all the aminoglycosides are similar. Therefore, one may consider gentamicin a model for the aminoglycosides in general, and the pharmacokinetic principles discussed in this chapter may be applied to other aminoglycosides as well. However, since the doses and therapeutic plasma concentrations differ among each of the agents, these values should be inserted into the appropriate equations.

Therapeutic and Toxic Plasma Concentrations

Peak plasma gentamicin concentrations of 4 to 8 mcg/ml (mg/L) are generally associated with clinical efficacy (79,80,81). Peak plasma concentrations less than 2 mcg/ml are likely to be ineffective (80), and successful treatment of pneumonia may require peak concentrations of 8 mcg/ml (79).

Almost all of the available data correlating gentamicin concentrations with oto- and nephrotoxicity refer to the trough plasma concentrations, although some data suggest a correlation of peak concentrations with toxicity (83,84). Because trough concentrations greater than 2 mcg/ml have been associated with renal toxicity, it has been suggested that this trough concentration not be exceeded (82). It is possible, however, that increased trough concentrations may be the result and not the cause of renal failure. The use of increased trough levels as an indication of early renal damage has been suggested by others (85). Fortunately, most patients who develop renal dysfunction during gentamicin therapy appear to regain normal renal function after discontinuation of the drug (90).

Ototoxicity has been associated with trough plasma concentrations exceeding 4 mcg/ml for more than 10 days. Most of the patients developing ototoxicity also had impaired renal function or had received large total doses of an aminoglycoside during the course of their treatment (83,84,85,86,89).

Volume of Distribution

The volume of distribution of gentamicin is usually reported to be approximately 0.25 L/kg, although a relatively wide range of 0.1 to 0.5 L/kg has been reported (91,92,93,94,95,96,107). The use of lean rather than total body weight will result in a more accurate approximation of Vd in obese patients (97). Others have suggested that the aminoglycoside volume of distribution in obese patients should be based on the patient's ideal body weight plus 50% of their excess weight (224,225).

A one compartment model is generally assumed for gentamicin pharmacokinetic calculations. However, an initial distribution phase occurs when gentamicin is administered by rapid intravenous infusion (98,99,100). For this reason, plasma samples obtained at the end of infusions lasting less than one hour may be higher than expected, and probably have no correlation with the therapeutic or toxic effects of the drug.

KEY PARAMETERS	
Therapeutic Plasma Concentrations	
Peak 4–8 mcg/ml (mg/L)	
Trough <2 mcg/ml (mg/L)	
Vd	0.25 L/kg
Cl	
Normal renal function	Equal to Cl_{Cr}
Anephric patients	2.5 ml/min (0.15 L/hr)
$\beta t_{1/2}$	2–5 hours

A third volume of distribution or gamma phase has been identified by Schentag et al (101). Because this final volume of distribution is large, and perhaps because of decreased gentamicin clearance when plasma levels are low, the average half-life associated with this third compartment is about 112 hours (98,101). This large final volume of distribution and long terminal half-life may be of significance in evaluating a patient's potential for gentamicin toxicity (102).

Despite the existence of three compartments for the volume of distribution of gentamicin, for clinical purposes it is sufficient to base pharmacokinetic calculations solely upon the second volume of distribution of 0.25 L/kg. When using the second volume of distribution exclusively, one should only evaluate concentrations greater than 1 mcg/ml. Furthermore, all plasma levels must be measured from samples obtained after the initial distribution phase. Generally, peak concentrations should be obtained one hour after the start of a maintenance dose, assuming the infusion period does not exceed one hour.

Clearance

Gentamicin is eliminated almost entirely by the renal route (96). Since gentamicin and creatinine clearances are similar over a wide range of renal function when gentamicin levels are within the therapeutic range (91,96,98), gentamicin clearance can be estimated from the formulas for creatinine clearance:

$$Cl_{Cr} \text{ for males (ml/min/70 kg)} = \frac{98 - 0.8(\text{age} - 20)}{SrCr} \qquad (\text{Eq. } 45)$$

$$Cl_{Cr} \text{ for females (ml/min/70 kg)} = 0.9 \left[\frac{98 - 0.8(\text{age} - 20)}{SrCr} \right] \qquad (\text{Eq. } 46)$$

Elimination Half-life

The elimination of gentamicin from the body is dependent upon its Vd and renal clearance. Since renal function varies considerably among individuals, the half-life varies considerably. For example, a 70 kg 25-year-old male with a serum creatinine of 0.8

mg/dl might have a gentamicin clearance of 117.5 ml/min (7.05 L/hr) which, assuming a volume of distribution of 0.25 L/kg, corresponds to an elimination half-life of 1.72 hours. On the other hand, a 75-year-old male with a similar volume of distribution and a serum creatinine of 1.4 mg/dl might have a gentamicin clearance of 38.6 ml/min (2.31 L/hr) and a half-life of 5.25 hours.

Nomograms

The wide availability of nomograms for the dosing of gentamicin may lead one to question the necessity of pharmacokinetic calculations for this drug (86). However, these nomograms are designed to achieve fixed peak and trough plasma concentrations and do not allow the clinician to individualize the dosage regimen with respect to the type of infection being treated or the benefit/risk ratio in the patient. Furthermore, nomograms are based upon average pharmacokinetic parameters and usually do not provide a method for dose adjustment based on observed plasma concentrations. An understanding of the basic pharmacokinetic principles as applied to gentamicin, coupled with a rational clinical approach, should provide optimal therapy for the less-than-average patient.

1. R.W. is a 30-year-old 70 kg woman with a serum creatinine of 0.8 mg/dl. She is given an initial gentamicin dose of 100 mg by intravenous infusion over one hour. Calculate the plasma concentration of gentamicin at the conclusion of the infusion.

By treating the infusion as a loading dose, a rough estimate of the gentamicin concentration at the end of a 100 mg infusion given over one hour can be obtained by dividing the administered dose of 100 mg by the volume of distribution. This method entails the use of a rearranged version of the loading dose equation. (Also see Part One, section on Selecting the Appropriate Equation). If a volume of distribution for gentamicin of 0.25 L/kg is assumed (91,97,107), R.W.'s volume of distribution is 17.5 L (0.25 L/kg × 70 kg). S and F are both 1.0.

$$\text{Loading Dose} = \frac{(Vd)(Cp)}{(S)(F)} \qquad \text{(Eq. 10)}$$

$$Cp^0 = \frac{(S)(F)(Dose)}{Vd} \qquad \text{(Eq. 40)}$$

$$= \frac{(1.0)(1.0)(100 \text{ mg})}{17.5 \text{ L}}$$

$$= 5.7 \text{ mg/L (mcg/ml)}$$

This approach makes two assumptions: [1] that we are working with a one compartment model, and [2] that the infusion was given quickly enough so that no significant elimination took place during the time of administration. The assumption of a one compartment model is appropriate for infusions lasting one hour. However, this assumption may not be valid when shorter infusion periods are used, because the duration of the infusion is insufficient to allow complete distribution to take place and the measured level at the end of the infusion may be higher than predicted (95,96,99).

The second assumption can be tested by calculating the expected half-life of gentamicin and comparing it with the duration of the infusion.

Since half-life is determined by volume of distribution and clearance, the patient's gentamicin clearance must first be estimated. Assuming gentamicin clearance is equal to creatinine clearance (96), this can be accomplished by estimating the creatinine clearance:

$$Cl_{Cr} \text{ (women, ml/min/70 kg)} = 0.9 \left[\frac{98 - 0.8(age - 20)}{SrCr} \right] \qquad \text{(Eq. 46)}$$

$$= 0.9 \left[\frac{98 - 0.8(30 - 20)}{0.8} \right]$$

$$= 0.9 \left[\frac{98 - 8}{0.8} \right]$$

$$= 101 \text{ ml/min}$$

Converting this gentamicin clearance to L/hr:

$$\frac{(101 \text{ ml/min})(60 \text{ min/hr})}{1000 \text{ ml/min}} = 6.06 \text{ L/hr}$$

This clearance value can now be used to calculate the half-life of gentamicin in this patient:

$$t\frac{1}{2} = \frac{(0.693)(Vd)}{Cl} \qquad \text{(Eq. 28)}$$

$$= \frac{(0.693)(17.5 \text{ L})}{6 \text{ L/hr}}$$

$$= 2 \text{ hours}$$

Since the infusion period of one hour is not substantially shorter than R.W.'s calculated half-life of two hours, significant elimination took place during the infusion and the second assumption does not hold. For this reason, one could assume that the calculated Cp^0 would be a high estimate of the measured Cp^0. Also see Part One, section on Clinical Application of Kd and Half-life: Dosing Interval.

2. Since R.W.'s loading dose infusion does not meet the two assumptions required to accurately estimate the initial drug plasma concentration (Cp^0) using Eq. 40, describe a more precise method of estimating this value.

R.W.'s situation is more accurately described by the equation for an infusion which is discontinued prior to steady state (Also see Part One, sections on Clinical Application of Kd and Half-life and Selecting of the Appropriate Equation):

$$Cp = \frac{(S)(F)(Dose/\alpha)}{Cl} \times (1 - e^{-Kdt_1}) \qquad \text{(Eq. 32)}$$

where τ is one hour since the 100 mg dose is infused over one hour, and t_1 is also one hour since we are solving for the plasma concentration at the end of the infusion period. The elimination rate constant (Kd) can be determined from the half-life (using Eq. 27) or directly from the clearance and volume of distribution (using Eq. 23):

$$Kd = \frac{0.693}{t\frac{1}{2}} \qquad \text{(Eq. 27)}$$

$$= \frac{0.693}{2 \text{ hr}}$$

$$= 0.34 \text{ hr}^{-1}$$

$$Kd = \frac{Cl}{Vd} \qquad\qquad \text{(Eq. 23)}$$

$$= \frac{6 \text{ L/hr}}{17.5 \text{ L}}$$

$$= 0.34 \text{ hr}^{-1}$$

If S and F are assumed to be 1.0, the peak concentration at the end of the one hour infusion can now be calculated:

$$Cp = \frac{(S)(F)(Dose/\tau)}{Cl} \times (1 - e^{-Kdt_1}) \qquad\qquad \text{(Eq. 32)}$$

$$= \frac{(1.0)(1.0)(100 \text{ mg/1 hr})}{6 \text{ L/hr}} \times (1 - e^{-(0.34/hr)(1 \text{ hr})})$$

$$= (16.6 \text{ mg/L})(1 - 0.71)$$

$$= (16.6 \text{ mg/L})(0.29)$$

$$= 4.8 \text{ mg/L}$$

This second estimate of 4.8 mg/L is somewhat less than the first estimate of 5.7 mg/L since it includes a correction for drug lost during the period of the infusion.

3. When would predictions of Cp^0 using the loading dose equations approximate those obtained through use of the infusion equation? See Questions 1 and 2.

Since the difference between the results obtained from these two approaches is the amount of drug cleared from the body during the infusion period, it would be reasonable to assume that in patients with a decreased gentamicin clearance either approach would be satisfactory. Since gentamicin is cleared renally, patients with significant renal failure could be handled either way.

4. Assume that the patient described in Question 1 (R.W.) is given 100 mg of gentamicin over 30 minutes. Estimate the plasma concentration 30 minutes after the completion of the infusion. Also assume that the drug behaves as though it were distributed into a single compartment.

A graphical representation of the plasma level versus time curve which would be produced by this situation would be similar to that depicted in Part One, Fig. 23: an infusion which is initiated and discontinued prior to the achievement of steady state. It is therefore appropriate to use Eq. 35 to estimate the gentamicin plasma concentration requested.

$$\text{Cp at } t_2 = \frac{(S)(F)(\text{Dose}/\tau)}{Cl} \times (1 - e^{-Kdt_1}) \times (e^{-Kdt_2}) \qquad \text{(Eq. 35)}$$

In this case τ and t_1 are 0.5 hours since that is the duration of the infusion, and t_2 is also 0.5 hours since that is the period of the plasma concentration decay after completion of the infusion. Again assuming S and F to be 1.0 and Kd, Vd and Cl to be 0.34 hr^{-1}, 17.5 L and 6 L/hr respectively,

$$Cp = \left[\frac{(1.0)(1.0)(100 \text{ mg}/0.5 \text{ hr})}{6 \text{ L/hr}} \right] [1 - e^{-(0.34)(0.5)}][e^{-(0.34)(0.5)}]$$

$$= \left[\frac{200 \text{ mg/hr}}{6 \text{ L/hr}} \right] [1 - e^{-0.17}][e^{-0.17}]$$

$$= (33.3 \text{ mg/L})(1 - 0.844)(0.844)$$

$$= (5.2 \text{ mg/L})(0.844)$$

$$= 4.4 \text{ mg/L (mcg/ml)}$$

An actual plasma sample taken at the end of the 30 minute infusion might be greater than the expected 5.2 mg/L because of incomplete distribution.

5. R.W., the 70 kg woman described in Question 1, was given 100 mg of gentamicin over one hour every eight hours. Predict her peak and trough plasma concentrations at steady state.

Again we could treat this regimen as though the patient were receiving intermittent intravenous boluses or as though she were receiving one hour infusions every eight hours. If the bolus model were applied, Eq. 36 could be used to predict the peak levels and Eq. 38 and 39 could be used to predict the trough levels (Also see Part One, section on Maximum and Minimum Plasma Concentrations):

$$\text{Cpss max} = \frac{\dfrac{(S)(F)(\text{Dose})}{Vd}}{(1 - e^{-Kd\tau})} \qquad \text{(Eq. 36)}$$

$$\text{Cpss min} = (\text{Cpss max})(e^{-Kd\tau}) \qquad \text{(Eq. 38)}$$

$$\text{Cpss min} = \frac{\dfrac{(S)(F)(Dose)}{Vd}}{(1-e^{-Kd\tau})} \times (e^{-Kd\tau}) \qquad \text{(Eq. 39)}$$

If we wish to use the infusion model, we would simply replace the term

$$\frac{(S)(F)(Dose)}{Vd}$$

in Eq. 36 and 39 with a term which describes the plasma concentration that can be expected at the conclusion of each infusion (Also see Part One, section on Clinical Application of Kd and Half-life):

$$\frac{(S)(F)(Dose/\tau)}{Cl} \times (1-e^{-Kdt_1})$$

where τ and t_1 are the time over which the infusion is administered. Since τ and t_1 are equal, they can both be referred to as $t_{infusion}$ or t_{in}. Now, substituting this infusion term into the equations for Cpss max and Cpss min (Eq. 36, 38 and 39), we have:

$$\text{Cpss max} = \frac{\dfrac{(S)(F)(Dose/t_{in})}{Cl} \times (1-e^{-Kdt_{in}})}{(1-e^{-Kd\tau})} \qquad \text{(Eq. 53)}$$

$$\text{Cpss min} = \text{Cpss max} \times e^{-Kd(\tau-t_{in})} \qquad \text{(Eq. 54)}$$

$$\text{Cpss min} = \frac{\dfrac{(S)(F)(Dose/t_{in})}{Cl} \times (1-e^{Kdt_{in}})}{(1-e^{-Kd\tau})} \times e^{-Kd(\tau-t_{in})} \qquad \text{(Eq. 55)}$$

which represent the peak and trough plasma levels following the infusion of a dose for t_{in} hour and repeated with a dosing interval of τ hours. See Fig. 1.

Assuming S and F are 1.0, the infusion time (t_{in}) is one hour, the dosing interval (τ) is eight hours, the clearance (Cl) is 6 L/hr and the elimination rate constant (Kd) is 0.34 hr^{-1}, the peak concentration at steady state would be calculated as follows:

$$\text{Cpss max} = \frac{\left[\dfrac{(1.0)(1.0)(100 \text{ mg/hr})}{6 \text{ L/hr}}\right][1 - e^{-(0.34)(1.0)}]}{1 - e^{-(0.34)(8)}}$$

$$= \frac{(16.6 \text{ mg/L})(1 - 0.71)}{1 - e^{-2.72}}$$

$$= \frac{(16.6 \text{ mg/L})(0.29)}{1 - 0.066}$$

$$= \frac{4.8 \text{ mg/L}}{0.934}$$

$$= 5.2 \text{ mg/L}$$

And the trough concentration would be:

$$\text{Cpss min} = \text{Cpss max} \times [e^{-Kd(\tau - t_{in})}] \qquad \text{(Eq. 54)}$$

$$= [5.2 \text{ mg/L}][e^{-(0.34)(8-1)}]$$

$$= (5.2 \text{ mg/L})(e^{-2.38})$$

$$= (5.2 \text{ mg/L})(0.093)$$

$$= 0.5 \text{ mg/L}$$

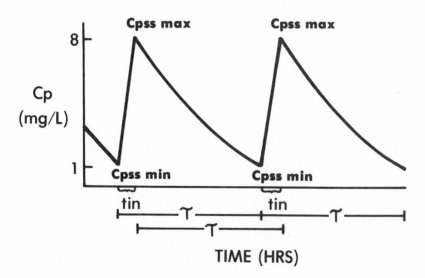

Fig. 1. Intermittent Intravenous Infusion at Steady State. The infusion is administered over t_{in} hours and τ is the dosing interval.

6. When gentamicin is administered by the intramuscular route, how should the steady state peak and trough plasma concentrations be calculated?

Although the time for peak plasma concentration following an intramuscular injection is variable, the majority of patients experience peak gentamicin concentrations after about one hour (80,96,98). Because of the potential problems in estimating the rate of absorption from the I.M. site, this situation can be approached as though it were an intravenous infusion taking place over a period of one hour. See Question 5.

7. L.K., a 40-year-old 50 kg female with a serum creatinine of 1 mg/dl, is to be given gentamicin. Calculate a maintenance dose which will achieve a peak concentration of 7 mg/L (mcg/ml) and a trough concentration of less than 2 mg/ L. Assume that the drug will be administered by infusion over one hour.

To calculate a maintenance dose which meets these objectives, one would rearrange the formula for Cpss max (Eq. 53) to solve for dose:

$$\text{Cpss max} = \frac{\dfrac{(S)(F)(\text{Dose}/t_{in})}{Cl} \times (1 - e^{-Kdt_{in}})}{(1 - e^{-Kd\tau})} \qquad \text{(Eq. 53)}$$

$$\text{Dose} = \frac{\text{Cpss max } (1 - e^{-Kd\tau})}{\dfrac{(S)(F)(1/t_{in})}{Cl} (1 - e^{Kdt_{in}})}$$

Before this equation can be solved, one must first calculate L.K.'s volume of distribution, clearance and elimination rate constant for gentamicin. A usual dosing interval of 8 hours will be assumed and adjusted later if necessary.

The volume of distribution of gentamicin in L.K. should be approximately 12.5 L if a Vd value of 0.25 L/kg is used.

The gentamicin clearance will be equal to L.K.'s creatinine clearance which can be calculated using Eq. 46:

$$Cl_{Cr} = 0.9 \left[\frac{98 - 0.8(\text{Age} - 20)}{\text{SrCr}} \right] \qquad \text{(Eq. 46)}$$

$$Cl_{Cr} = 0.9 \left[\frac{98 - 0.8(40 - 20)}{1 \text{ mg/dl}} \right]$$

$$= 74 \text{ ml/min/70 kg or } 4.44 \text{ L/hr}$$

The calculated clearance of 4.44 L/hr/70kg should be adjusted to L.K.'s weight of 50 kg (Body surface area may also be used):

$$\text{Patient's Clearance} = \text{Calculated Clearance} \times \frac{\text{Patient's weight}}{70 \text{ kg}}$$

$$= 4.44 \text{ L/hr} \times \frac{50 \text{ kg}}{70 \text{ kg}}$$

$$= 3.17 \text{ L/hr}$$

The elimination rate constant can be calculated using equation 23:

$$Kd = \frac{Cl}{Vd} \qquad \text{(Eq. 23)}$$

$$= \frac{3.17 \text{ L/hr}}{12.5 \text{ L}}$$

$$= 0.25 \text{ hr}^{-1}$$

Using the rearranged version of the Equation for Cpss max (see above), the dose which would produce a maximum concentration of 7 mg/L would be 87.3 mg administered over one hour every 8 hours:

$$\text{Dose} = \frac{7 \text{ mg/L} \left(1 - e^{-0.25 \text{ hr}^{-1} \times 8 \text{ hr}}\right)}{\dfrac{(1)(1)(1/1 \text{ hr})}{3.17 \text{ L/hr}} \left(1 - e^{-0.25 \text{ hr}^{-1} \times 1 \text{ hr}}\right)}$$

$$= \frac{6}{0.315 \times 0.22}$$

$$= 87.3$$

The trough concentration which will be produced by this dosage regimen can be calculated using Eq. 54:

$$\text{Cpss min} = \text{Cpss max} \times e^{-Kd(\tau - t_{in})} \qquad \text{(Eq. 54)}$$

$$= 7 \text{ mg/L} \times e^{-0.25 \text{ hr}^{-1}(8 \text{ hr} - 1 \text{ hr})}$$

$$= 1.2 \text{ mg/L}$$

The trough concentration of 1.2 mg/L is below the desired maximum trough concentration of 2 mg/L. If the trough level had been above 2 mg/L, the dosing interval would have to be increased and a new dose calculated by using the rearranged version of Eq. 53.

8. Y.B., a 70 kg 38-year-old patient with a serum creatinine of 1 mg/dl, has been receiving 100 mg of gentamicin over one hour every eight hours for several days. A peak plasma concentration obtained at the end of the infusion was 5.2 mcg/ml (mg/L) and a trough concentration obtained just before the start of the next infusion was 1.0 mcg/ml (mg/L). Estimate the apparent elimination rate constant (Kd), clearance, and volume of distribution for gentamicin in Y.B.

The two reported plasma concentrations were measured from samples obtained during the elimination phase of the plasma concentration versus time curve. Since the 7 hour time interval between samples exceeds the half-life of gentamicin in this patient, the two concentrations can be used to estimate the elimination rate constant, Kd. See Part One, section on Elimination Rate Constant and Eq. 24:

$$Kd = \frac{\ln\left[\frac{Cp_1}{Cp_2}\right]}{t} \qquad (Eq.\ 24)$$

$$= \frac{\ln\left[\frac{5.2}{1.0}\right]}{7\ hrs}$$

$$= \frac{1.65}{7\ hrs}$$

$$= 0.235\ hrs^{-1}$$

Since all of the troughs are equal at steady state (see Part One, Fig. 25), the same samples could have been obtained immediately prior to and after the same infusion. If this had been done as a matter of convenience, the interval between samples would still be considered to be seven hours because the trough value obtained just prior to the infusion would actually represent the level just prior to the subsequent infusion.

Using the elimination rate constant of 0.235 hr^{-1}, the observed Cpss max of 5.2 mg/L and the dosage regimen of 100 mg/hr, the patient's clearance can be calculated by rearranging Eq. 53.

$$\text{Cpss max} = \frac{\dfrac{(S)(F)(\text{Dose}/t_{in})}{Cl} \times (1 - e^{-Kdt_{in}})}{1 - e^{-Kd\tau}} \qquad \text{(Eq. 53)}$$

$$Cl = \frac{\dfrac{(S)(F)(\text{Dose}/t_{in})}{\text{Cpss max}} \times (1 - e^{-Kdt_{in}})}{1 - e^{-Kd\tau}}$$

$$= \frac{\dfrac{(1.0)(1.0)(100 \text{ mg/hr})}{5.2 \text{ mg/L}} \times [1 - e^{-(0.235)(1)}]}{1 - e^{-(0.235)(8)}}$$

$$= \frac{(19.23 \text{ L/hr})(1 - 0.79)}{1 - 0.153}$$

$$= \frac{(19.23 \text{ L/hr})(0.21)}{0.847}$$

$$= 4.77 \text{ L/hr}$$

Since the clearance and the elimination rate constant are now known, Eq. 23 can be rearranged to calculate the apparent volume of distribution:

$$Kd = \frac{Cl}{Vd} \qquad \text{(Eq. 23)}$$

$$Vd = \frac{Cl}{Kd}$$

$$= \frac{4.77 \text{ L/hr}}{0.235 \text{ hr}^{-1}}$$

$$= 20.3 \text{ L}$$

This volume of distribution would correspond to about 0.29 L/kg.

The value of calculating gentamicin pharmacokinetic parameters which are specific for Y.B. is that they may be used to calculate a dosing regimen that will produce any desired peak and trough concentration.

These parameters which are based on observed plasma concentrations are somewhat different than would be predicted given the patient's age, weight and serum creatinine, but they are not so unusual as to be considered unreasonable. If the calculations had led to parameters that were very different from those that were expected, it may indicate an error in the time of sampling, the assay or the dosing history. In such cases it may be more prudent to use the expected rather than calculated parameters. However, there is always the possibility that a patient really does have unusual parameters, and in such cases it is wise to re-evaluate the history and obtain another set of plasma drug concentrations, being certain as to the exact time of sampling and the dosing history.

9. D.L., a 38-year-old 70 kg patient with renal failure, is receiving gentamicin and carbenicillin for treatment of a fever of unknown origin. How might the concurrent administration of carbenicillin influence the pharmacokinetics of gentamicin? Are there other antibiotic combinations that may influence gentamicin dosing?

The beta-lactam ring of penicillin compounds interacts with gentamicin both *in vivo* and *in vitro* to form an inactive amide (103,105). However, the rate of this inactivation is slow and it only contributes significantly to the elimination of gentamicin in patients with severely impaired renal function (104,105,106). In these patients, the concurrent administration of carbenicillin can decrease the half-life of gentamicin from 46 to 22 hours. It has been recommended that the two antibiotics be administered separately and that the dose of carbenicillin be decreased in such cases. An alternative may be to substitute gentamicin with amikacin which appears to be more resistant to degradation by penicillin than other aminoglycosides (103).

The combination of cephalosporins and aminoglycosides may place patients at greater risk for nephrotoxicity (108,109).

10. What is the significance of a changing serum creatinine in a patient receiving gentamicin?

A rising serum creatinine in a patient must always raise the question of gentamicin-induced nephrotoxicity. In this event, the drug should be discontinued, the plasma concentration evaluated, and the dose adjusted since gentamicin may accumulate substantially when renal function is impaired. Dosage modifications should be based upon plasma gentamicin levels rather than serum creatinine levels, since serum creatinine concentrations which are not at steady state can be misleading.

Despite the similarity of gentamicin and creatinine clearances (96,98), their volumes of distribution differ (gentamicin's Vd of 0.25 L/kg is smaller than that of creatinine–0.4 to 0.6 L/kg) (12,24,91,92,107). Since the half-life is determined by the clearance and volume of distribution (see Eq. 28 below), the half-life for creatinine is longer than gentamicin's and it will take longer to arrive at a new steady state after a change in renal function.

$$t\frac{1}{2} = \frac{0.693Vd}{Cl} \qquad \text{(Eq. 28)}$$

When the serum creatinine is rising (i.e. not at steady state), renal function is worse than would be predicted by the serum creatinine and any gentamicin dosage calculated using a serum creatinine would be overestimated. Conversely, when the serum creatinine is falling, renal function may be better than that reflected by the serum creatinine and doses calculated on the basis of these levels would be underestimated.

11. D.W. is a 20-year-old, 60 kg male patient receiving 80 mg of gentamicin (as a 1 hour infusion) every 8 hours. His serum creatinine has increased from 1 to 2 mg/dl over the past 24 hours indicating a sudden decrease in his renal function. Because of his increasing serum creatinine three samples were drawn: one just prior to a dose; one, 1 hour after the same dose; and one 8 hours after the dose (two troughs and one peak level). These levels were reported as 4 mg/L, 8 mg/L, and 5 mg/L respectively. Calculate the volume of distribution, elimination rate constant and clearance of gentamicin in D.W.

Since the second trough concentration of gentamicin is higher than the first, it is apparent that the drug is accumulating; therefore, steady state equations should not be used in the calculation of the patient's pharmacokinetic parameters.

Volume of Distribution. If D.W.'s renal clearance of gentamicin is low, it is reasonable to assume that little drug will be eliminated during the one hour infusion and to calculate the apparent volume of distribution using a variation of Eq. 10, the loading dose equation (Also see Question 3). Since the concentration produced by the dose is the difference between the peak and trough concentration, Cp in the equation will be equal to 4 mg/L:

$$\text{Loading Dose} = \frac{(Vd)(Cp)}{(S)(F)} \qquad \text{(Eq. 10)}$$

$$= (Vd)(Cp) \text{ when S and F are 1.0.}$$

therefore,

$$Vd = \frac{\text{Loading Dose}}{Cp}$$

$$= \frac{80 \text{ mg}}{(8 \text{ mg/L} - 4 \text{ mg/L})}$$

$$= 20 \text{ L}$$

Elimination Rate Constant. Since we have two plasma concentrations which were obtained during the elimination phase of the concentration versus time curve (8 mg/L and 5 mg/L), Eq. 24 can be used to estimate the elimination rate constant. However, this Kd should only be used as an estimate since the two plasma concentrations were obtained less than one half-life ($\approx$ 12 hr in this patient) apart.

$$Kd = \frac{\ln\left(\dfrac{Cp_1}{Cp_2}\right)}{t} \qquad \text{(Eq. 24)}$$

$$= \frac{\ln\left(\dfrac{8 \text{ mg/L}}{5 \text{ mg/L}}\right)}{8 \text{ hr}}$$

$$= 0.059 \text{ hr}^{-1}$$

$$t\frac{1}{2} = \frac{0.693}{Kd}$$

$$= \frac{0.693}{0.059 \text{ hr}^{-1}}$$

$$= 11.7 \text{ hr}$$

Clearance. The clearance can be calculated from the volume of distribution and elimination rate constant using Eq. 29:

$$Cl = (Kd)(Vd) \qquad \text{(Eq. 29)}$$

$$= 0.059 \ hr^{-1} \times 20 \ L$$

$$= 1.18 \ L/hr \ or \ 19.6 \ ml/min$$

Note that this clearance is considerably less than that which would have been predicted using the nonsteady state serum creatinine concentration of 2 mg/dl obtained at the time the gentamicin levels were drawn.

12. Using the pharmacokinetic parameters calculated for D.W. in Question 11, develop a dosing regimen which will produce reasonable peak and trough concentrations.

Since D.W.'s gentamicin clearance is low (1.18 L/hr), it will be necessary to reduce his maintenance dose. There are two alternatives: reduce the dose and maintain the same dosing interval or adjust both the dose and dosing interval such that the peak and trough concentrations will be approximately 8 mg/L and 2 mg/L respectively.

Reduce the dose and maintain the same dosing interval. This method is not acceptable in this patient because he has such a long half-life ($\approx$ 12 hours). If a dose which achieves a Cpss max of 8 mg/L is used and the dosing interval of 8 hours is maintained, the trough level would be approximately 5 mg/L. This level may place the patient at greater risk for gentamicin toxicity:

$$Cpss \ min = (Cpss \ max) \times (e^{-Kdr}) \qquad \text{(Eq. 38)}$$

$$= (8 \ mg \ L) \times (e^{-0.059/hr \times 8 \ hr})$$

$$= 5 \ mg/L$$

Adjust both the dose and dosing interval to achieve reasonable peak and trough concentrations. The only limitation to this approach is that most clinicians like to avoid prolonged periods of time during which the gentamicin concentration is below 1 or 2 mg/L because of the possibility of breakthrough bacteremia. Generally, if a compromise must be made, one should tolerate a trough concentration which is slightly higher than ideal to minimize the risk of therapeutic failure. This is despite the fact that there are some animal data which suggest that high peak and low trough concentrations produce less renal toxicity than that produced by the same dose administered as an intravenous infusion (i.e., the same average levels) (88).

A first estimate of the dosing interval can be made by examining the gentamicin half-life. If a dose which produces a peak concentration of 8 mg/L is selected, it is clear that a trough concentration of 2 mg/L will be produced after two half-lives. Therefore a dosing interval of 24 hours can be used. The dose which will produce a Cpss max of 8 mg/L can be calculated using a rearranged version of the Cpss max equation for a "bolus" infusion (Eq. 53) as in Question 7. However, because this patient has such a long gentamicin half-life, it is satisfactory to use the intravenous bolus model or Eq. 36:

$$\text{Cpss max} = \frac{(S)(F)(\text{Dose})/Vd}{1 - e^{-Kd\tau}} \qquad \text{(Eq. 36)}$$

$$\text{Dose} = \frac{\text{Cpss max} \times (1 - e^{-Kd\tau}) \times Vd}{(S)(F)}$$

$$= \frac{8 \text{ mg/L} \times (1 - e^{0.05 \, 9/hr \times 24 \, hr}) \times 20 \text{ L}}{(1)(1)}$$

$$= 121 \text{ mg every 24 hours}$$

The trough concentration produced by this dose would be 1.9 mg/L (see Eq. 38):

$$\text{Cpss min} = (\text{Cpss max})(e^{Kd\tau}) \qquad \text{(Eq. 38)}$$

$$= (8 \text{ mg/L})(e^{-0.059/hr \times 24 \, hr})$$

$$= 1.9 \text{ mg/L}$$

If a higher trough concentration is desired, the dosing interval would be shortened and a new dose would be calculated.

13. M.S. is a 70 kg patient receiving hemodialysis every 48 hours. She is surgically anephric and is to be started on

gentamicin. Calculate a dosing regimen which will achieve and then maintain peak concentrations of 6 mg/L.

Since very little gentamicin will be cleared during the infusion, the loading dose may be calculated as though it were a bolus. Assuming S and F to be 1.0 and the volume of distribution to be 17.5 L (0.25 L/kg), the loading dose would be calculated as follows:

$$\text{Loading Dose} = \frac{(Vd)(Cp)}{(S)(F)} \qquad \text{(Eq. 10)}$$

$$= \frac{(17.5 \text{ L})(6 \text{ mg/L})}{(1.0)(1.0)}$$

$$= 105 \text{ mg}$$

Since the clearance will be irregular, occurring at a higher rate during the dialysis period, the usual maintenance dose equation would not be appropriate. Instead, the problem should be approached by evaluating the drug loss between and during the dialysis periods and giving an appropriate replacement dose. Assuming that the loading dose were given immediately after dialysis, the plasma concentration after 48 hours could be calculated using Equation 22:

$$Cp = (Cp^0)(e^{-Kdt}) \qquad \text{(Eq. 22)}$$

In order to use this equation, the elimination rate constant must be known. This can be determined from the reported clearance of gentamicin in surgically anephric patients, which is about 2.5 ml/min or 0.15 L/hr (92,110). Using this clearance and the assumed volume of distribution of 17.5 L, the elimination rate constant can be calculated:

$$Kd = \frac{Cl}{Vd} \qquad \text{(Eq. 23)}$$

$$= \frac{0.15 \text{ L/hr}}{17.5 \text{ L}}$$

$$= 0.0086 \text{ hr}^{-1}$$

Eq. 22 can now be used to predict the gentamicin level after 48 hours of decay:

$$Cp = (Cp^0)(e^{-Kdt}) \qquad\qquad\qquad\qquad \text{(Eq. 22)}$$

$$= (6\ \mathrm{mg/L})(e^{-(0.0086)(48)})$$

$$= (6\ \mathrm{mg/L})(e^{-0.41})$$

$$= (6\ \mathrm{mg/L})(0.664)$$

$$= 4\ \mathrm{mg/L}$$

Therefore, the plasma concentration just before dialysis would be 4 mg/ml. Most studies indicate that the clearance of aminoglycosides by hemodialysis is about 20 to 40 ml/min (92,110,111,114). Using the most frequently quoted value of 25 ml/min and adding it to the residual nonrenal clearance of 2.5 ml/min, the total clearance while on dialysis is about 1.65 L/hr:

$$\frac{(25\ \mathrm{ml/min} + 2.5\ \mathrm{ml/min})(60\ \mathrm{min/hr})}{1000\ \mathrm{ml/L}} = 1.65\ \mathrm{L/hr}$$

This clearance and the volume of distribution of 17.5 L result in a gentamicin half-life estimate of about 7.3 hours and an elimination rate constant of 0.095 hr^{-1} while on dialysis:

$$t\tfrac{1}{2} = \frac{0.693 Vd}{Cl} \qquad\qquad\qquad\qquad \text{(Eq. 28)}$$

$$= \frac{0.693(17.5\ \mathrm{L})}{1.65\ \mathrm{L/hr}}$$

$$= 7.3\ \mathrm{hours}$$

$$Kd = \frac{0.693}{t\tfrac{1}{2}}$$

$$= \frac{0.693}{7.3\ \mathrm{hr}}$$

$$= 0.095\ \mathrm{hr}^{-1}$$

Since the usual dialysis time is 6 to 8 hours, one would expect the plasma gentamicin concentration to decline by about one-half because the patient is being dialyzed for one half-life. Therefore, at the end of the dialysis the gentamicin concentration should have declined from 4 to about 2 mg/L. A more specific concentration at the end of dialysis could be calculated from Eq. 22 using the new Kd value and the time of dialysis.

At this point an additional dose should be given to again achieve a peak concentration of 6 mg/L. Since there is a residual plasma concentration, Eq. 11 should be used to calculate the next loading dose:

$$\text{Loading Dose} = \frac{(Vd)(Cp \text{ desired} - Cp \text{ initial})}{(S)(F)} \quad \text{(Eq. 11)}$$

$$= \frac{(17.5 \text{ L})(6 \text{ mg/L} - 2 \text{ mg/L})}{(1.0)(1.0)}$$

$$= 70 \text{ mg}$$

If there had been any residual renal function, it would have been added to the assumed nonrenal clearance of 2.5 ml/min (92). If the patient had also been receiving carbenicillin or other penicillin-type antibiotic, the expected gentamicin half-life would be much shorter than would be predicted from any residual renal and assumed nonrenal clearance (105,106).

Unfortunately, the persistence of relatively high plasma concentrations between dialysis periods will place this patient at greater risk for developing vestibular toxicity (112).

14. How would the above situation have differed if peritoneal dialysis were being used rather than hemodialysis?

Peritoneal dialysis is much less efficient in removing gentamicin; the usual clearance values are between 5 and 10 ml/min. Nevertheless, the total amount of drug removed during dialysis may be as much as 30% or more because peritoneal dialysis is usually continued for about 36 hours (110,113).

15. A patient with meningitis is being considered for treatment with intrathecal or intraventricular gentamicin. Which of these routes is preferred and what pharmacokinetic parameters would be expected?

Gentamicin does not cross the blood-brain barrier very efficiently and CSF levels are usually subtherapeutic unless intrathecal or intraventricular injections are given (115,116). The intraventricular route is preferred in order to insure adequate ventricular levels and a uniform concentration throughout the subarachnoid space (115). Intraventricular gentamicin doses of 5 to 10 mg usually result in CSF levels of 12 to 40 mcg/ml or higher for the first six hours after the injection; CSF levels decline to approximately 5 mcg/ml after 24 hours (115). The apparent cerebrospinal fluid half-life of gentamicin is approximately six hours (115,116). The dose of 5 to 10 mg is usually repeated on a daily basis. If the intraventricular route is to be used, a special access port or shunt would have to be installed.

8

Phenobarbital

Phenobarbital is a long-acting barbiturate which is used in the treatment of seizure disorders and, because of its sedative-hypnotic properties, as an "anti-anxiety" agent. It is most commonly administered orally, but it may be administered intramuscularly and intravenously as well.

The usual adult maintenance dose of 2 mg/kg/day will produce a steady state plasma concentration of approximately 20 mcg/ml. Because phenobarbital has a half-life of 5 days, therapeutic plasma concentrations are not achieved for two or three weeks following the initiation of a maintenance regimen. When therapeutic levels of 20 mcg/ml are required immediately, a loading dose of 15 mg/kg can be administered.

Therapeutic Concentrations

In adults, phenobarbital concentrations of 10–30 mcg/ml are required for seizure control (142). The upper end of the therapeutic range is limited by the appearance of side effects such as central nervous system depression and ataxia (143), although occasional patients exhibit no symptoms of toxicity even with phenobarbital concentrations in excess of 40 mcg/ml (144). Phenobarbital concentrations in excess of 100 to 150 mcg/ml are considered potentially lethal, although patients with much higher concentrations have survived (144,145,146).

Bioavailability

While it has not been well studied, the data available indicate that at least 80% and probably greater than 90% of phenobarbital administered orally is absorbed. Complete bioavailability is supported by the observation that similar plasma concentrations result when the same dose of phenobarbital is given orally and parenterally.

KEY PARAMETERS	
Therapeutic Concentrations	10–30 mcg/ml
Bioavailability (F)	>0.9
S (for Na salt)	0.9
Vd	0.6–0.7 L/kg
Cl[a]	4 ml/hr/kg (0.096 L/day/kg)
t½	5 days

[a] Primarily metabolized by the liver. 20% cleared renally.

Phenobarbital is frequently administered as the sodium salt which is 91% phenobarbital acid (S = 0.91); however, a correction for the salt form is seldom made since the degree of error is small and the therapeutic range is relatively broad.

Volume of Distribution

The volume of distribution for phenobarbital is approximately 0.6 to 0.7 L/kg (147,148).

Clearance

Phenobarbital is primarily metabolized by the liver; less than 20% is eliminated by the renal route (151). The average total plasma clearance for phenobarbital is approximately 4 ml/hr/kg or 0.096 L/day/kg.

Half-life

The plasma half-life of phenobarbital is 5 days.

1. W.R., a 39-year-old 70 kg male, developed grand mal seizures several months after an automobile accident in which he sustained head injuries. Phenobarbital is to be initiated in this patient. Calculate a loading dose of phenobarbital that will produce a plasma level of 20 mcg/ml (mg/ L).

Since this is a loading dose problem in which there is no existing initial drug concentration, Eq. 10 should be used:

$$\text{Loading Dose} = \frac{(Vd)(Cp)}{(S)(F)} \qquad \text{(Eq. 10)}$$

If F and S are assumed to be 1.0 and the volume of distribution is assumed to be 0.7 L/kg or 49 L, the expected loading dose will be 980 mg or approximately 1 gm:

$$\text{Loading Dose} = \frac{(49\ \text{L})(20\ \text{mg/L})}{(1.0)(1.0)}$$

$$= 980\ \text{mg}$$

$$\approx 1\ \text{gm}$$

This 1 gm dose is very close to the usual loading dose of 15 mg/kg. It may be administered orally, intramuscularly or intravenously.

Generally, the loading dose is divided into three or more portions and administered over several hours. The necessity for dividing the loading dose is not entirely clear; it is probably done as a precaution against toxicity should two compartment distribution exist or to avoid cardiovascular toxicity from the propylene glycol diluent in the injectable dosage form (see Phenytoin chapter).

2. Calculate an oral maintenance dose for W.R. which will maintain a phenobarbital concentration of 20 mcg/ml. How should the dose be administered?

Since clearance is the major determinant of the maintenance dose, this parameter must be estimated for W.R. While there is some intersubject variability, the average clearance of phenobarbital in adults is 4 ml/hr/kg or 0.096 L/day/kg. Thus, the expected clearance for W.R., who is 70 kg, is 6.72 L/day:

$$\text{Clearance} = 0.096\ \text{L/day/kg} \times 70\ \text{kg}$$

$$= 6.72\ \text{L/day}$$

If S and F are assumed to be 1.0, the maintenance dose of phenobarbital can be calculated using Eq. 15:

$$\text{Maintenance Dose} = \frac{(Cl)(Cpss\ ave)(\tau)}{(S)(F)} \qquad \text{(Eq. 15)}$$

$$= \frac{(6.7\ 2\ L/day)(20\ mg/L)(1\ day)}{(1.0)(1.0)}$$

$$= 134\ mg$$

In practice, the daily dose is usually divided into two or more portions; however, with a half-life of 5 days, once daily dosing should suffice (147):

$$t\frac{1}{2} = \frac{(0.693)(Vd)}{Cl} \qquad \text{(Eq. 28)}$$

$$= \frac{(0.693)(49\ L)}{6.72\ L/day}$$

$$= 5\ days$$

Interestingly, the calculated dose corresponds closely to an empiric clinical guideline which has been used for many years: The phenobarbital steady state level (in mcg/ml) produced by any given maintenance dose will be approximately equal to ten times the daily dose in mg/kg:

$$\text{W.R.'s Maintenance Dose (mg/kg)} = \frac{134\ mg}{70\ kg}$$

$$= 1.9\ mg/kg$$

According to the clinical guideline, the level in mcg/ml produced by this dose will be 19 mcg/ml (1.9 × 10). This level is very close to the desired Cpss ave level of 20 mcg/ml.

3. If W.R. does not receive a loading dose, how long will it take to achieve a minimum therapeutic level of 10 mcg/ml following the initiation of the maintenance dose? How long will it take to achieve a steady state level of 20 mcg/ml?

To answer a question involving time, a knowledge of the half-life is required. The half-life for phenobarbital in this patient is 5 days as calculated in Question 2. If it takes three to five half-lives to reach steady state, approximately 15 to 20 days will be required to achieve the final plateau concentration of 20 mcg/ml. See Part One, Fig. 17.

Since 10 mcg/ml is one-half the steady state value, it will take one half-life or 5 days to reach this level. That is, one-half of steady state is achieved in the first half-life.

4. K.P., a 62-year-old 57 kg female patient, was admitted for poor seizure control. Prior to admission she had been receiving an unknown dose of phenobarbital. On admission, the phenobarbital concentration was 5 mcg/ml, and she was started on 60 mg of phenobarbital every 8 hours. Five days later, the phenobarbital concentration was measured and reported as 17 mcg/ml. Calculate her final steady state concentration on the present regimen.

There are several ways of approaching this problem. Since Cpss ave is defined by clearance, one could use the average clearance for phenobarbital (0.096 L/day/kg × 57 kg = 5.5 L/day) and insert this value into Eq. 31:

$$\text{Cpss ave} = \frac{(S)(F)(\text{Dose}/\tau)}{Cl} \qquad \text{(Eq. 31)}$$

$$= \frac{(1)(1)(180 \text{ mg/day})}{5.5 \text{ L/day}}$$

$$= 33 \text{ mg/L or mcg/ml}$$

Another method which could be used to estimate the steady state value is as follows. Assume that the concentration of 17 mcg/ml reported on the 5th day represents the sum of the fraction of the initial concentration (5 mcg/ml) remaining at this point in time plus the accumulated concentration resulting from five daily doses of 180 mg. If this patient's half-life for phenobarbital is 5 days, the fraction of the initial concentration remaining after one half-life will be 0.5 and contribution to the reported concentration at 5 days will be 2.5 mcg/ml. The remaining portion of the reported concentration (14.5 mcg/ml) represents 50% of the steady state level which will be produced by the 180 mg/day dose. Therefore, the predicted Cpss ave would be 29 mcg/ml (2 × 14.5 mcg/ml).

One could also use the empiric clinical guideline discussed in Question 3 regarding the prediction of Cpss ave from the mg/kg dose of phenobarbital. In this case the mg/kg dose would be 180 mg/57 kg or 3.16 mg/kg. The predicted Cpss ave would be 31.6 mcg/ml (3.16 × 10).

All of these estimates are based upon the assumption that the patient's pharmacokinetic parameters for phenobarbital are similar to those reported in the literature. Since the estimates for Cpss ave are at the high end of the therapeutic range, it would be reasonable to obtain another plasma concentration 15 to 20 days after the initiation of the maintenance dose. Also, because the repeat concentration will be obtained after more than one half-life has passed, the patient's parameters for phenobarbital can be estimated more reliably. (See Theophylline chapter, Questions 11 and 12).

5. J.R., an epileptic who has been managed chronically on phenobarbital 120 mg/day, has recently developed hypoalbuminemia secondary to nephrotic syndrome. Will his phenobarbital concentration be affected by his albumin concentration or renal function?

Only 40 to 50% of phenobarbital is bound to plasma proteins; therefore, alpha or the fraction of phenobarbital which is free is 0.5 to 0.6 (153,154). The concentrations of drugs which are bound to proteins to the extent of 50% or less are not likely to be significantly affected by changes in plasma protein concentrations or protein binding affinity.

The renal clearance for phenobarbital is probably less than 20% of the total clearance in patients whose urine flow is normal and whose urine pH is uncontrolled (that is, the urine pH is not being intentionally adjusted through the administration of drugs) (151). Therefore, it is unlikely that patients with renal failure will require significant adjustments in their phenobarbital dosage regimens.

To summarize, J.R.'s phenobarbital concentrations are not likely to be affected by his hypoalbuminemia or poor renal function.

6. R.T. is a 25-year-old, 70 kg patient with chronic renal failure and a seizure disorder. He has been maintained on

60 mg of phenobarbital twice daily and has steady state concentrations of 20 mg/ml. Over the past three months, his renal failure has become progressively worse and he is to be started on 6 hours of hemodialysis three times a week. Will he require an adjustment of his maintenance regimen?

To determine whether or not a significant amount of drug is lost during each dialysis session, one must determine the fraction of drug remaining (and thereby lost) during the six hour period. See Eq. 22:

$$Cp = (Cp^0)(e^{-Kdt}) \tag{Eq. 22}$$

where Cp^0 and Cp are the phenobarbital concentrations at the beginning and end of the dialysis period, t is the duration of dialysis and e^{-Kdt} is the fraction of the initial concentration remaining at the end of six hours of dialysis.

The Kd for phenobarbital during dialysis can be calculated from the dialysis clearance of phenobarbital. The clearance of phenobarbital by hemodialysis has not been studied extensively; however, there are two reports on the use of hemodialysis in the treatment of patients intoxicated with phenobarbital which indicate that the hemodialysis clearance is about 3.5 L/hr (3 to 4 L/hr) (146,152). If this value is inserted into Eq. 23, Kd can be derived.

$$Kd = \frac{Cl}{Vd} \tag{Eq. 23}$$
$$= \frac{3.5 \text{ L/hr}}{49 \text{ L}}$$
$$= 0.071 \text{ hr}^{-1}$$

Then, by inserting this Kd value into Eq. 22, the concentration of phenobarbital remaining at the end of each dialysis (assuming $Cp^0 = 20$ mcg/ml) will be 13 mcg/ml and the concentration which was lost during that same period will be 7 mcg/ml (20 mcg/ml − 13 mcg/ml).

The dose which will replace the amount of phenobarbital lost during the dialysis can be calculated by multiplying the concentration lost by the patient's volume of distribution for phenobarbital, 49 L.

$$\text{Loading Dose} = \frac{(Vd)(Cp)}{(S)(F)} \hspace{3cm} \text{(Eq. 10)}$$

$$= \frac{(7 \text{ mg/L})(49 \text{ L})}{(1)(1)}$$

$$= 343 \text{ mg or approximately } 350 \text{ mg}$$

This post dialysis replacement dose should be administered in addition to the usual maintenance dose, since the patient's metabolic clearance is ongoing and was not considered in the determination of phenobarbital clearance during the dialysis period.

9

Phenytoin

Phenytoin is primarily used as an anticonvulsant and is occasionally used in the treatment in certain types of cardiac arrhythmia (199). It is usually administered orally in single or divided doses of 200 to 400 mg per day. When a rapid therapeutic effect is required, a loading lose of 15 mg/kg can be administered by the oral or intravenous route. Although approved for use, the intramuscular route should be avoided because of slow and erratic absorption.

The use of phenytoin in the clinical setting has two major problems. First, phenytoin binds extensively to plasma proteins. This binding is decreased in patients with renal failure or hypoalbuminemia, making therapeutic and pharmacokinetic interpretation difficult. Second, the metabolic capacity for phenytoin is limited so that modest changes in the maintenance dose result in disproportionate changes in the steady state plasma concentration.

Therapeutic and Toxic Plasma Concentrations

Phenytoin plasma concentrations of 10 to 20 mcg/ml (mg/L) are generally accepted as therapeutic. Plasma concentrations in the range of 5 to 10 mcg/ml can be therapeutic for some patients, but concentrations below 5 mcg/ml are not likely to be effective.

A number of phenytoin side effects, such as gingival hyperplasia, folate deficiency and peripheral neuropathy, do not appear to be related to plasma phenytoin concentrations. In contrast, central nervous system (CNS) side effects do correlate with plasma concentration. Far-lateral nystagmus is probably the most common CNS side effect and usually occurs in patients with plasma phenytoin concentrations greater then 20 mcg/ml. However, the concentration range associated with this side effect is broad, with some patients showing symptoms at concentrations of 15 mcg/ml and others having no nystagmus with concentrations greater than 30

KEY PARAMETERS	
Therapeutic Concentrations	10 to 20 mcg/ml (mg/L)
Bioavailability (F)	1.0
Vd	0.65 L/kg
Cl	Concentration dependent
Vm	7 mg/kg/day
Km	4 mg/L
t½	Concentration dependent
α (fraction free in plasma)	0.1

mcg/ml. Other CNS symptoms such as ataxia and diminished
mental capacity are frequently observed in patients with concentrations exceeding 30 and 40 mcg/ml respectively (202). In addition, precautions should be taken when phenytoin is administered
by the intravenous route, as the propylene glycol diluent has
cardiac depressant properties (200).

Bioavailability

The bioavailability of phenytoin is difficult to evaluate because
of the drug's capacity limited metabolism. It appears that phenytoin is completely absorbed (F = 1.0) from most products currently
available (230). There is a difference in the salt form, however.
The capsules and injectable preparation are the sodium salt (S
= 0.92), while the chewable tablets and suspension are the acid
form (S = 1.0). Due to the limited solubility of phenytoin, the rate
of absorption following oral administration is slow, with peak
concentrations occurring three to 12 hours after administration
(197).

Volume of Distribution

The volume of distribution of phenytoin in patients with normal
renal function and serum albumin is approximately 0.65 L/kg
(40,147,196).

Capacity Limited Metabolism

For most drugs the rate of metabolism (and/or excretion) is
governed by the plasma concentration. Clearance is the volume of
plasma which is completely cleared of drug per unit of time (see

Part One, section on Clearance). Throughout this text we have used equations in which clearance is the fixed proportionality constant which makes the steady state plasma concentration equal to the rate of drug administration (R_A):

$$R_A = (Cl)(Cpss\ ave)$$
(Eq. 13)

where R_A is $(S)(F)(Dose/\tau)$. However, *this usual case of first-order kinetics does not apply to phenytoin,* in that the clearance decreases as Cpss ave increases.

The clearance of phenytoin from plasma occurs primarily by metabolism, and the rate of this drug's metabolism approaches its maximum at therapeutic concentrations. Thus, *the metabolism of phenytoin is described as being capacity limited* (196,202–206). Capacity limited metabolism results in clearance values that decrease with increasing plasma concentrations. This implies that as the maintenance dose is increased, the plasma concentration rises disproportionately (203,207–212) (See Fig. 1). This disproportionate rise in the steady state plasma level makes dosage adjustment more difficult than with first-order drugs which have a constant clearance and a steady state plasma concentration which is proportional to the maintenance dose.

The model which appears to fit the metabolic pattern for phenytoin elimination is the one originally proposed by Michaelis and Menten. The velocity (v) or rate at which an enzyme system can metabolize a substrate (s) can be described by the following equation:

$$v = \frac{(Vm)(s)}{Km + s}$$
(Eq. 56)

where Vm is the maximum metabolic capacity and Km is the substrate concentration at which v will be one half of Vm. This relationship has been applied successfully to phenytoin by substituting the average steady state phenytoin concentration (Cpss ave) for s and the daily dose or administration rate of phenytoin $[R_A$ or $(S)(F)(Dose/\tau)]$ for v (208,210,211,212). When these substitutions are made, Eq. 56 can be rewritten as:

$$(S)(F)(Dose/\tau) = \frac{(Vm)(Cpss)}{Km + Cpss}$$
(Eq. 57)

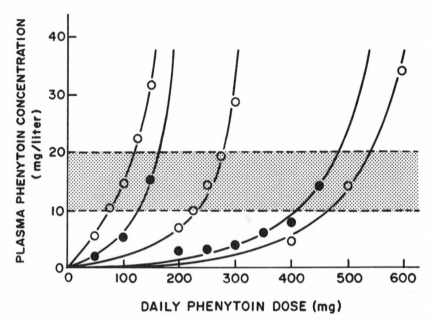

Fig. 1. For each patient the plasma phenytoin concentration at steady state increases disproportionately with an increase in the rate of administration. In all patients the daily dose required to achieve a steady state concentration of 20 mg/L is not much greater than that required to achieve a value of 10 mg/L, the therapeutic concentration range. The five patients were selected in this study because their dosage needed to be changed several times to control their epileptic seizures. Figure modified from that in reference 231.

Eq. 57 can also be rearranged as follows:

$$\text{Cpss} = \frac{\text{Km} \times (\text{S})(\text{F})(\text{Dose}/\tau)}{\text{Vm} - (\text{S})(\text{F})(\text{Dose}/\tau)}$$ (Eq. 58)

In accordance with the original definition of Vm and Km for Eq. 56, Vm is the maximum rate of metabolism (metabolic capacity) and Km is the plasma concentration at which the rate of metabolism is one half the maximum. The units for Vm and Km are mg/day and mg/L, respectively.

Equation 58 illustrates the sensitive relationship between the rate of phenytoin administration and Cpss when the rate of administration approaches Vm, the maximum metabolic capacity. The rate of phenytoin administration must be less than Vm or steady state will never be achieved. If Vm minus $(S)(F)(Dose/\tau)$ were 0, Cpss would be infinity:

$$Cpss = \frac{Km \times (S)(F)(Dose/\tau)}{Vm - (S)(F)(Dose/\tau)} \tag{Eq. 58}$$

$$= \frac{Km \times (S)(F)(Dose/\tau)}{0}$$

$$= \infty$$

The range of plasma concentrations which have been reported to result in a metabolic rate which is one half the maximum (Km) is between 1 and more than 20 mg/L (mcg/ml) (207,209,210,211,213). The maximum metabolic capacity (Vm) appears to be between 5 and 15 mg/kg/day in most patients (207,210,211). The relationship between Km and Vm is not clear, but it appears that if one of these parameters is low, the other is also usually low (207,208,211). The average values of Km and Vm have not been established. It is the author's opinion that 4 mg/L for Km and 7 mg/kg/day for Vm are reasonable estimates for the average patient.

Concentration Dependent Clearance. When $(S)(F)(Dose/\tau)$ from Eq. 14, the usual equation for clearance, is substituted into Eq. 57 a new equation for clearance can be obtained:

$$Cl = \frac{(S)(F)(Dose/\tau)}{Cpss\ ave} \tag{Eq. 14}$$

can be rearranged to:

$$(S)(F)(Dose/\tau) = Cl \times Cpss\ ave$$

and substituted into Eq. 57:

$$(S)(F)(Dose/\tau) = \frac{(Vm)(Cpss)}{Km + Cpss} \tag{Eq. 57}$$

$$Cl = \frac{Vm}{Km + Cpss} \tag{Eq. 59}$$

Since clearance is dependent on concentration, this expression of clearance has little utility and probably should never be used. However, the equation points out the relationship between phenytoin concentration (Cpss) and clearance. If Cpss is very small compared to Km, clearance will be a relatively constant value of Vm/Km and the metabolism will appear to be first order. When Cpss approaches or exceeds Km, the apparent clearance will decrease and the metabolism will no longer appear to be a first-order process. As clearance decreases with increasing phenytoin concentration, the velocity or metabolic rate will also increase, but *not* in proportion to the increase in plasma concentration (see Fig. 1). Because Km is below the usual therapeutic range, nearly all patients will display capacity limited metabolism.

Concentration Dependent Half-Life. The usual reported half-life for phenytoin is approximately 22 hours (204), but one would not expect the half-life to be constant since clearance changes with the plasma concentration. If Eq. 59 (the clearance equation for phenytoin) is substituted into Eq. 28 (the usual equation for half-life), the half-life of phenytoin can be derived:

$$Cl = \frac{Vm}{Km + Cpss} \tag{Eq. 59}$$

$$t\frac{1}{2} = \frac{(0.693)(Vd)}{Cl} \tag{Eq. 28}$$

$$t\frac{1}{2} = \left(\frac{(0.693)(Vd)}{Vm}\right)(Km + Cpss) \tag{Eq. 60}$$

Based on Eq. 60 it can be predicted that the half-life of phenytoin will increase as the plasma concentration increases, an observation that has been confirmed (205).

The utility of the phenytoin half-life is limited in that the time required to achieve steady state can be much longer than three to four of the apparent half-lives. Likewise, the time required for a plasma concentration to decay following discontinuation of the maintenance dose will be less than predicted by the apparent half-life.

1. Calculate the phenytoin loading dose required to achieve a plasma concentration of 20 mcg/ml (mg/L) in a 70 kg patient.

Assuming that phenytoin has a volume of distribution of 0.65

L/kg, the volume of distribution for a 70 kg patient would be 45.5 L (70 kg × 0.65 L/kg). If the phenytoin is administered as capsules or as the injectable form, S will be 0.92 since the sodium salt is used in both of these dosage forms. Assuming the bioavailability to be 100% (F = 1.0), Eq. 10 can be used to estimate the loading dose that will achieve a plasma concentration of 20 mcg/ml (mg/L):

$$\text{Loading Dose} = \frac{(Vd)(Cp)}{(S)(F)} \quad\quad \text{(Eq. 10)}$$

$$= \frac{(45.5\ L)(20\ mg/L)}{(0.92)(1.0)}$$

$$= 989\ mg$$

This loading dose of 989 mg is reasonably close to the usual, recommended loading dose of 1000 mg. If this dose is administered intravenously, it should be administered slowly to avoid the cardiovascular toxicities associated with the propylene glycol diluent (200). A maximum rate of 50 mg/min or 100 mg every 5 minutes should be used until the entire loading dose is administered or toxicities are encountered (199). If the 1000 mg loading dose is to be given orally, it has been suggested that a 400 mg dose followed by two 300 mg doses at two-hour intervals be administered so that the entire loading dose is administered over 4 hours. The oral dose is divided to avoid nausea and vomiting which is associated with a single 1 gm dose (201). When the loading dose is administered orally, slow absorption causes the peak concentration to be delayed and lower than the expected 20 mg/L (201).

2. S.B. is a 68.5 kg, 37-year-old male with a seizure disorder which has only partially been controlled with 300 mg/day of phenytoin. His plasma phenytoin concentration has been measured twice over the past year and both times it was reported to be 7.0 mcg/ml (mg/L). Calculate a dose which will achieve a steady state concentration of 14 mcg/ml (mg/L).

To establish the new daily dose, it is necessary to assume a Vm or Km for S.B. and then rearrange Eq. 57 to calculate the other parameter. Rearranging Eq. 57 to solve for Vm,

$$(S)(F)(Dose/\tau) = \frac{(Vm)(Cpss)}{Km + Cpss} \qquad \text{(Eq. 57)}$$

$$Vm = \frac{(S)(F)(Dose/\tau)(Km + Cpss)}{Cpss} \qquad \text{(Eq. 61)}$$

If Km is assumed to be 4 mg/L, S to be 0.92 (capsules contain the sodium salt) and F to be 1.0, then Vm would be:

$$Vm = \frac{(0.92)(1.0)(300 \text{ mg/day})(4 \text{ mg/L} + 7 \text{ mg/L})}{7 \text{ mg/L}}$$

$$= \frac{(276 \text{ mg/day})(11 \text{ mg/L})}{7 \text{ mg/L}}$$

$$= 434 \text{ mg/day}$$

To calculate the dose required to achieve a steady state concentration of 14 mg/L, Eq. 57 can be rearranged as follows:

$$(S)(F)(Dose/\tau) = \frac{(Vm)(Cpss)}{Km + Cpss} \qquad \text{(Eq. 57)}$$

$$Dose = \frac{(Vm)(Cpss)(\tau)}{(Km + Cpss)(S)(F)} \qquad \text{(Eq. 62)}$$

Using the assumed Km of 4 mg/L and the calculated Vm of 434 mg/day, the daily dose required to achieve a steady state of 14 mg/L would be:

$$Dose = \frac{(434 \text{ mg/day})(14 \text{ mg/L})(1 \text{ day})}{(4 \text{ mg/L} + 14 \text{ mg/L})(0.92)(1.0)}$$

$$= 367 \text{ mg}$$

This dosage adjustment of 22% should result in a 100% increase in the steady state plasma level if our assumed Km of 4 mg/L is correct. Because a daily dose of 367 mg would be difficult to administer, this initial dosing estimate would probably be rounded off to 350 mg/day, which could be achieved by having the patient take 300 and 400 mg on alternate days.

3. Calculate an appropriate loading dose that would rapidly increase S.B.'s plasma phenytoin concentration from 7 to 14 mg/L.

Assuming a volume of distribution of 44.5 L (68.5 kg × 0.65 L/kg), S = 0.92 and F = 1.0, the loading dose required to increase S.B.'s plasma concentration from 7 to 14 mg/L would be:

$$\text{Loading Dose} = \frac{(Vd)(Cp\ desired - Cp\ initial)}{(S)(F)} \quad \text{(Eq. 11)}$$

$$= \frac{(44.5\ L)(14\ mg/L - 7\ mg/L)}{(0.92)(1.0)}$$

$$= 338\ mg$$

This loading dose should be given in addition to the new maintenance dose of 350 mg/day. It may be appropriate to divide the dose in order to avoid the gastrointestinal side effects that have been reported with single large doses of phenytoin (201).

Administration of the loading dose will allow more rapid evaluation of the new maintenance dose. If the plasma concentration is less than 14 mg/L after one week, a second dosage adjustment can be made at that time. If a loading dose is not given and at the end of one week the plasma concentration is less than 14 mg/L, one could not determine whether or not steady state concentrations had been achieved.

4. R.M. is a 32-year-old, 80 kg male who is being seen in the Neurology Clinic. Prior to his last visit he had been taking 300 mg of phenytoin daily; however, because his seizures were poorly controlled and because his plasma concentration was only 8 mg/L, his dose was increased to 350 mg/daily. Now he complains of minor CNS side effects and his reported plasma phenytoin concentration is 20 mg/L. Renal and hepatic function are normal. Assume that both of the reported plasma concentrations represent steady state and that the patient has complied with the prescribed dosing regimens. Calculate R.M.'s apparent Vm and Km and a new daily dose of phenytoin that will result in a steady state level of about 15 mg/L.

The relationship between daily dose and Cpss can be made linear by plotting daily dose (rate in) *versus* daily dose divided by Cpss (clearance) for at least two steady state plasma levels. The graph for R.M. is plotted in Fig. 2, where the rate in intercept (390 mg/day) is Vm and the slope of the line (-2.5 mg/L) is the negative value of Km.

Using these values, the daily dose of phenytoin which will achieve a steady state level of 15 mg/L can be calculated as follows:

$$\text{Dose} = \frac{(\text{Vm})(\text{Cpss})(\tau)}{(\text{Km} + \text{Cpss})(\text{S})(\text{F})} \qquad \text{(Eq. 62)}$$

$$= \frac{(390 \text{ mg/day})(15 \text{ mg/L})(1 \text{ day})}{(2.5 \text{ mg/L} + 15 \text{ mg/L})(1.0)(1.0)}$$

$$= 334 \text{ mg}$$

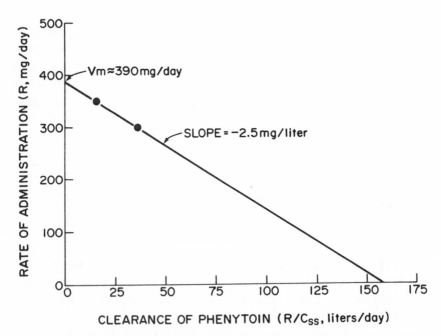

Fig. 2. **The Rate of Administration (R) or the Daily Dose of Phenytoin (mg/day) Versus the Clearance of Phenytoin (R/Cpss, L/day) is Plotted for Two or More Different Daily Doses of Phenytoin.** A straight line of the best fit is drawn through the points plotted. The intercept on the rate of administration axis is Vm (mg/day) and the slope of the line is the negative value of Km:

$$\text{Slope} = \frac{R_1 - R_2}{\left(\dfrac{R_1}{\text{Cpss}_1}\right) - \left(\dfrac{R_2}{\text{Cpss}_2}\right)}$$

The closest convenient dose to the calculated value of 334 mg/day would be 330 mg/day, which could be administered as three 100 mg capsules and one 30 mg capsule.

S was assumed to be 1.0 in the above equation, despite the fact that R.M. is taking phenytoin capsules which contain the sodium salt. Compensation for salt form would be inappropriate since the actual doses of phenytoin sodium were plotted in Fig. 2. If the doses had been plotted as phenytoin acid, the Vm would have been slightly lower, Km would have been unchanged, and an S of 0.92 would have been used in Eq. 62 to calculate the daily dose required to achieve a steady state concentration of 15 mg/L.

5. If R.M.'s doses are withheld, how long will it take for the phenytoin concentration of 20 mg/L to decline to 15 mg/ L?

As stated earlier, the phenytoin half-life will be of little value in predicting the time required for the plasma concentration to decay, because the apparent half-life will change as the plasma concentration changes.

The time required for the phenytoin plasma concentration to fall from an initial concentration (Cp^0) to a lower concentration (Cp) can be expressed as follows:

$$t = \frac{Km \times \ln\left(\frac{Cp^0}{Cp}\right) + (Cp^0 - Cp)}{\dfrac{Vm}{Vd}} \qquad \text{(Eq. 63)}$$

For R.M., who has a volume of distribution of 52 L (0.65 L/kg × 80 kg), a Vm of 390 mg/day and a Km of 2.5 mg/L, the time required for the initial plasma concentration of 20 mg/L to decline to 15 mg/L will be about 0.76 days:

$$t = \frac{2.5 \text{ mg/L} \times \ln\left(\frac{20}{15}\right) + (20 \text{ mg/L} - 15 \text{ mg/L})}{\dfrac{390 \text{ mg/day}}{52 \text{ L}}}$$

$$= \frac{(2.5 \text{ mg/L} \times 0.288) + 5 \text{ mg/L}}{7.5 \text{ mg/day/L}}$$

$$= 0.76 \text{ days}$$

This rate of decline assumes that phenytoin will not continue to be absorbed from the GI tract for a significant period following discontinuation of the drug. In practice, however, the initial rate of decline is slower than expected because of prolonged absorption (Author's observation).

6. E.W. is a 56-year-old 60 kg woman who has chronic renal failure and a seizure disorder. She receives hemodialysis three times a week and takes 300 mg of phenytoin daily. Her reported steady state plasma phenytoin concentration is 5 mcg/ml. Should her daily phenytoin dose be increased? What would her phenytoin concentration be if she had normal renal function? (Assume her albumin concentration is normal.)

It is critical to carefully evaluate measured phenytoin concentrations in uremic patients because plasma protein binding is altered in these individuals. In patients with normal renal function, about 90% of the measured plasma phenytoin concentration is bound to albumin and 10% is free (α = 0.1) (5,40,214). Because of decreased binding affinity in uremia and because of decreased albumin concentration, the fraction of the total phenytoin concentration which is free in patients with very poor renal function increases from 0.1 to the range of 0.2 to 0.35 (20,40,215–217). In patients with renal failure who have normal serum albumin levels, the fraction free is approximately 0.2 (40,215). Also see Part One, Figs. 3 and 5 and section on Desired Plasma Concentration.

Since the fraction free (α) for phenytoin is increased in uremics, lower plasma concentrations will be required to achieve pharmacologic effects which are equivalent to those produced by higher levels in nonuremic individuals. E.W.'s case can be used to illustrate this principle.

Assuming that E.W.'s uremia has reduced the binding of her plasma phenytoin to 80% (20% free or α = 0.2), the free concentration produced by a measured plasma concentration of 5 mcg/ml can be calculated using Eq. 8:

$$\text{Cp free} = (\alpha)(\text{Cp total}) \qquad \text{(Eq. 8)}$$

$$= (0.2)(5 \text{ mcg/ml})$$

$$= 1.0 \text{ mcg/ml}$$

This free concentration of 1.0 mcg/ml produced by a measured plasma concentration of 5 mcg/ml in E.W. would be equivalent to the free concentration produced by a measured concentration of 10 mcg/ml in a patient with normal plasma protein binding. This is illustrated through a rearrangement of Eq. 8 to solve for Cp total. The known free concentration of 1.0 mcg/ml and an α for a nonuremic patient (0.1) are used to calculate the equivalent Cp total for a nonuremic individual.

$$\text{Cp free} = (\alpha)(\text{Cp total}) \qquad\qquad\qquad \text{(Eq. 8)}$$

can be arranged to solve for Cp total:

$$\text{Cp total} = \frac{\text{Cp free}}{\alpha}$$

$$\text{Cp total} = \frac{1.0 \text{ mcg/ml}}{0.1}$$

$$= 10 \text{ mcg/ml}$$

Therefore, E.W.'s measured plasma phenytoin concentration of 5 mcg/ml is comparable to a concentration of 10 mcg/ml in a patient with normal plasma binding. The usually accepted therapeutic range for phenytoin in nonuremic patients is 10 to 20 mcg/ml, and E.W.'s free plasma concentration corresponds to the low end of this range. If E.W.'s seizure disorder is well controlled, no adjustment in the maintenance dose is necessary. However, if seizures are poorly controlled and an adjustment is necessary, the comparable plasma concentration for a patient with normal plasma binding (10 mcg/ml) should be used in all calculations since the values for Km reported in the literature were determined in patients with normal plasma protein binding. Another approach would be to determine the Km appropriate to the degree of plasma protein binding. The important point is that whenever Km and Cp are used in an equation together, they should reflect the same alpha value.

Dialysis does not appear to significantly remove phenytoin or to change the binding characteristics of a uremic patient's protein (20,215). In addition, it is not known how much time is required for the change in plasma protein binding to occur once a patient develops acute renal failure. There is some evidence that following a renal transplant, the plasma protein binding for phenytoin increases rapidly over the first 2 to 4 post-operative days and is almost normal two weeks following a successful transplant (216).

7. S.T. is a 47-year-old 60 kg man with glomerular nephritis. His creatinine clearance is reasonably good, but he has a serum albumin of 2.0 gm/dl. S.T. is receiving 300 mg/day of phenytoin and has a steady state phenytoin concentration of 6 mcg/ml. What would his phenytoin concentration be if his serum albumin were normal? (Assume 4.0 gm/dl to be normal.)

The fraction of a drug concentration which is bound to plasma proteins is a function of drug affinity for the binding sites on the plasma protein (illustrated in the previous question) and the number of binding sites available. The number of binding sites is proportional to the amount or concentration of plasma protein to which the drug is bound. Phenytoin is an acidic drug and appears to be bound primarily to albumin (5). The relationship between a phenytoin concentration (Cp′) which is observed when a patient has a low serum albumin (P′) relative to the phenytoin concentration (Cp adjusted) which would be observed if the serum albumin were normal (P) is described by Eq. 6, and in its rearranged form by Eq. 7 (see Part One, section on Desired Plasma Concentration and Figs. 3,4,5):

$$\frac{Cp'}{Cp \text{ adjusted}} = (1-\alpha)\left(\frac{P'}{P}\right) + \alpha \qquad \text{(Eq. 6)}$$

$$Cp \text{ adjusted} = \frac{Cp'}{(1-\alpha)\left(\frac{P'}{P}\right) + \alpha} \qquad \text{(Eq. 7)}$$

The plasma phenytoin concentration that would correspond to a normal albumin concentration in S.W. can be calculated as follows:

$$Cp \text{ adjusted} = \frac{Cp'}{(1-\alpha)\left(\frac{P'}{P}\right) + \alpha} \qquad \text{(Eq. 7)}$$

$$= \frac{6 \text{ mcg/ml}}{(1-\alpha)\left(\frac{2.0 \text{ gm/dl}}{4.0 \text{ gm/dl}}\right) + 0.1}$$

$$= \frac{6 \text{ mcg/ml}}{(0.9 \times 0.5) + 0.1}$$

$$= 10.9 \text{ mcg/ml}$$

Cp adjusted should be used in any calculations requiring Km, as described in the previous question.

8. How would S.T.'s Cp adjusted have been affected if he were also in renal failure?

If S.T. were uremic in addition to having a low serum albumin, even lower plasma protein binding would result. When both renal failure and low serum albumin are present, Eq. 64 should be used to adjust for both of these factors:

$$\text{Cp adjusted} = \frac{\text{Cp}'}{\left[(1-\alpha)\left(0.44 \times \frac{\text{P}'}{\text{P}}\right)\right] + \alpha} \qquad \text{(Eq. 64)}$$

Again, Cp' is the observed phenytoin concentration, and Cp adjusted is the plasma concentration that would be seen if the serum albumin (P') were normal (P) and alpha were normal (0.1). The adjustment factor of 0.44 is an empiric value which assumes that alpha is 0.2 in uremic patients who have normal serum albumin levels. The relationship of phenytoin plasma protein binding to the degree of renal impairment is not known since most investigators studied patients with end stage renal failure. Therefore Eq. 64 applies only to patients with end stage renal failure.

9. A.R. is a 66-year-old, 60 kg patient who was admitted to the hospital because of poor seizure control. He had been receiving 350 mg/day of phenytoin acid as an outpatient and on admission had a plasma level of 3 mg/L. Noncompliance was suspected, and a dose of 350 mg per day was ordered. Five days after administration a second phenytoin level was reported as 18 mg/L. Has steady state been achieved? Is it reasonable to assume that A.R.'s values for Vm and Km are

close to the average values reported in the literature (i.e., Vm = 7 mg/kg/day and Km = 4 mg/L)?

Because the metabolism of phenytoin is capacity limited, the usual guideline which uses three to four half-lives to estimate the time required to achieve steady state does not hold true. The rate of phenytoin accumulation is the difference between the rate of metabolism and the rate of administration. However, unlike drugs following first-order elimination, the rate of elimination does not increase proportionately to the plasma concentrations. Therefore, the time required to reach steady state is much longer than would be predicted if the drug's accumulation and elimination followed a first-order process. The discrepancy between the expected time to reach steady state assuming a first-order process and the actual time to reach steady state is greatest when the plasma concentrations are much greater than Km. The following equation can be used to estimate the time (t) required to achieve 90% of steady state assuming the initial plasma phenytoin concentration is zero. Km, Vm and Vd are the assumed or derived parameters for the patient.

$$t_{90\%} = \frac{(Vm)(Vd)}{(Vm-R_A)^2}[2.303(Vm-0.9R_A)] \qquad \text{(Eq. 65)}$$

If the usual values for Vm (7 mg/kg/day) and Km (4 mg/L) are assumed for A.R., solution of Eq. 65 for $t_{90\%}$ results in an answer of 725 days. Since it actually took only 5 days for the plasma level to increase from 3 to 18 mg/L, the rate of accumulation is more rapid than expected. Therefore, it appears that A.R.'s rate of metabolism is slower than expected and that Vm and Km for A.R. are probably less than the average values reported in the literature. The use of this equation helps confirm original estimates and gives a more objective estimate of the time required for phenytoin accumulation.

10. Why does changing from oral to intramuscular phenytoin result in a sudden and dramatic decrease in phenytoin levels?

Phenytoin is a relatively insoluble compound which crystallizes within the muscle following intramuscular administration (222). It appears that the phenytoin crystals are slowly absorbed, resulting in an initial reduction in the phenytoin dosage (absorption) rate. In addition, because of capacity-limited phenytoin metabolism, the drop in plasma level will be more than proportional to the reduction in absorption from the intramuscular injection. This was well demonstrated by Wilder (223) when a change from oral to intramuscular administration resulted in an initial 40 to 60% decrease in the phenytoin plasma level, while the metabolite elimination decreased by only 16 to 20%. Because of the unpredictable absorption following intramuscular injection, this route of administration should be avoided.

11. What effect does phenobarbital have on steady state phenytoin concentrations? What other drugs might interact with phenytoin?

Clinically, the addition of phenobarbital does not change steady state phenytoin concentrations (218). However, it is possible that phenobarbital may induce the metabolism of phenytoin and thereby increase its metabolic capacity (increase Vm). Furthermore, competition between phenobarbital and phenytoin for the same enzymes would have the effect of increasing Km. The effect of increasing Vm would be to increase clearance and reduce the phenytoin concentration. Increasing Km would have the opposite effect; therefore, there may be no net effect on the phenytoin concentration.

$$Cpss = \frac{Km \times (S)(F)(Dose/\tau)}{Vm - (S)(F)(Dose/\tau)} \qquad \text{(Eq. 58)}$$

Similar problems exist in evaluating the mechanism for the increased phenytoin concentrations associated with drugs such as isoniazid and chloramphenicol (219,220). In the case of isoniazid, there are animal data which suggest the mechanism is a noncompetitive inhibition for metabolic enzymes which reduces the Vm (221). The interaction appears to be more significant in patients who are phenotypically slow acetylators of isoniazid (221).

Valproic acid, phenylbutazone, and salicylates have been reported to reduce the phenytoin concentration by displacement from albumin (231). This mechanism would decrease the total phenytoin concentration but not the free or unbound concentration. The result is an increased α and a decreased therapeutic range.

APPENDICES

NOMOGRAMS FOR CALCULATING BODY SURFACE AREA

Nomogram for Calculating the Body Surface Area of Children[1]

Height	Surface area	Weight

1) From the formula of DuBois and DuBois, *Arch. intern. Med.*, **17**, 863 (1916):

$$S = W^{0.425} \times H^{0.725} \times 71.84, \text{ or } \log S = 0.425 \log W + 0.725 \log H + 1.8564,$$

where S = body surface area in square centimeters, W = weight in kilograms, H = height in centimeters.

Nomogram for Calculating the Body Surface Area of Adults[1]

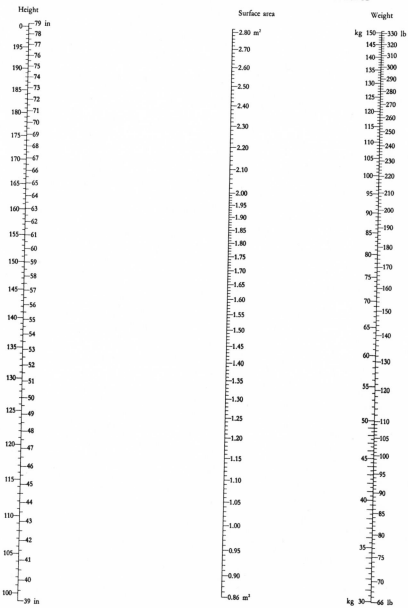

Height	Surface area	Weight

1) From the formula of DuBois and DuBois, *Arch. intern. Med.*, **17**, 863 (1916):

$S = W^{0.425} \times H^{0.725} \times 71.84$, or $\log S = 0.425 \log W + 0.725 \log H + 1.8564$,

where S = body surface area in square centimeters, W = weight in kilograms, H = height in centimeters.

APPENDIX II

EQUATIONS USED THROUGHOUT THE TEXT

The following is the list of equations as they are presented in the text. Although the list appears long and complicated, most of the equations can be broken down into one or more of the following four elements:

$\dfrac{(S)(F)(Dose)}{Vd}$ The change in plasma concentration following a dose.

$\dfrac{(S)(F)(Dose)}{(Cl)(\tau)}$ Average steady state concentration.

(e^{-Kdt}) Fraction remaining at the end of a decay phase.

$(1 - e^{-Kdt})$ Fraction lost during decay phase or fraction of steady state achieved during infusion.

$$(F)(Dose) = \text{Amt. of Drug Absorbed or} \atop \text{Amt. of Drug Reaching the Systemic Circulation} \qquad \text{(Eq. 1)}$$

$$\frac{\text{Dose of New}}{\text{Dosage Form}} = \frac{\begin{array}{c}\text{Amount of Drug Absorbed from}\\ \text{Current Dosage Form}\end{array}}{\text{F of New Dosage Form}} \qquad \text{(Eq. 2)}$$

$$(S)(F)(Dose) = \text{Amt. of Drug Absorbed or} \atop \text{Amt. Reaching the Systemic Circulation} \qquad \text{(Eq. 3)}$$

$$\frac{\text{Administration Rate}}{(R_A)} = \frac{(S)(F)(Dose)}{\tau} \qquad \text{(Eq. 4)}$$

$$\alpha = \frac{\text{Free drug concentration}}{\text{Total drug concentration}} = \frac{\text{Cp free}}{\text{Cp bound} + \text{Cp free}} \qquad \text{(Eq. 5)}$$

$$\frac{Cp'}{Cp \text{ adjusted}} = (1 - \alpha)\left(\frac{P'}{P}\right) + \alpha \qquad \text{(Eq. 6)}$$

$$\text{Cp adjusted} = \frac{\text{Cp}'}{(1-\alpha)\left(\dfrac{\text{P}'}{\text{P}}\right)+\alpha}$$ (Eq. 7)

$$\text{Cp free} = (\alpha)(\text{Cp total})$$ (Eq. 8)

$$\text{Vd} = \frac{\text{Ab}}{\text{Cp}}$$ (Eq. 9)

$$\text{Loading Dose} = \frac{(\text{Vd})(\text{Cp})}{(\text{S})(\text{F})}$$ (Eq. 10)

$$\text{Loading Dose} = \frac{(\text{Vd})(\text{Cp desired} - \text{Cp initial})}{(\text{S})(\text{F})}$$ (Eq. 11)

$$R_A = R_E$$ (Eq. 12)

$$R_A = (\text{Cl})(\text{Cpss ave})$$ (Eq. 13)

$$\text{Cl} = \frac{(\text{S})(\text{F})(\text{Dose}/\tau)}{\text{Cpss ave}}$$ (Eq. 14)

$$\text{Maintenance Dose} = \frac{(\text{Cl})(\text{Cpss ave})(\tau)}{(\text{S})(\text{F})}$$ (Eq. 15)

$$\text{BSA in m}^2 = \left(\frac{\text{Patient's weight in kg}}{70 \text{ kg}}\right)^{0.73}(1.73 \text{ m}^2)$$ (Eq. 16)

$$\text{Patient's Cl} = (\text{Literature Cl/70 kg})\left(\frac{\text{Patient's BSA}}{1.73 \text{ m}^2}\right)$$ (Eq. 17)

$$\text{Patient's Cl} = (\text{Literature Cl/70 kg})\left(\frac{\text{Patient's wt in kg}}{70 \text{ kg}}\right)$$ (Eq. 18)

$$\text{Patient's Cl} = (\text{Literature Cl/kg})(\text{Patient's wt in kg})$$ (Eq. 19)

$$\text{Cl}_t = \text{Cl}_m + \text{Cl}_r$$ (Eq. 20)

$$\text{Cl}_{\text{adjusted}} = \text{Cl}_m + \begin{array}{l}(\text{Cl}_r \times \text{Fraction of Normal Renal} \\ \text{Function Remaining})\end{array}$$ (Eq. 21)

$$\text{Cp} = (\text{Cp}^0)(e^{-\text{Kdt}}) \text{ or } \text{Ab} = (\text{Ab}^0)(e^{-\text{Kdt}})$$ (Eq. 22)

$$\text{Kd} = \frac{\text{Cl}}{\text{Vd}}$$ (Eq. 23)

$$Kd = \frac{\ln\left(\frac{Cp_1}{Cp_2}\right)}{t} \qquad \text{(Eq. 24)}$$

$$Kd_{adjusted} = K_{metabolic} + \left(K_{renal} \times \begin{array}{l}\text{Fraction of Normal}\\\text{Renal Function}\\\text{Remaining}\end{array}\right) \qquad \text{(Eq. 25)}$$

$$Cl_{adjusted} = (Kd_{adjusted} \times Vd_{normal}) \qquad \text{(Eq. 26)}$$

$$t\frac{1}{2} = \frac{0.693}{Kd} \qquad \text{(Eq. 27)}$$

$$t\frac{1}{2} = \frac{(0.693)(Vd)}{Cl} \qquad \text{(Eq. 28)}$$

$$Cl = (Kd)(Vd) \qquad \text{(Eq. 29)}$$

$$\begin{array}{l}\text{Fraction of Steady State}\\\text{Achieved at } t_1\end{array} = 1 - e^{-Kdt_1} \qquad \text{(Eq. 30)}$$

$$Cpss\ ave = \frac{(S)(F)(Dose/\tau)}{Cl} \qquad \text{(Eq. 31)}$$

$$\text{Plasma Concentration at } t_1 = \frac{(S)(F)(Dose/\tau)}{Cl} \times (1 - e^{-Kdt_1}) \qquad \text{(Eq. 32)}$$

$$Cpss\ ave = \frac{\text{Plasma Concentration at } t_1}{(1 - e^{-Kdt_1})} \qquad \text{(Eq. 33)}$$

$$\text{Fraction of Drug Remaining at } t_2 = (e^{-Kdt_2}) \qquad \text{(Eq. 34)}$$

$$\begin{array}{c}\text{Plasma Concentration}\\\text{at } t_2\end{array} = \frac{(S)(F)(Dose/\tau)}{Cl} \times (1 - e^{-Kdt_1})(e^{-Kdt_2}) \qquad \text{(Eq. 35)}$$

$$Cpss\ max = \frac{\dfrac{(S)(F)(Dose)}{Vd}}{(1 - e^{-Kd\tau})} \qquad \text{(Eq. 36)}$$

$$Cpss\ min = Cpss\ max - \frac{(S)(F)(Dose)}{Vd} \qquad \text{(Eq. 37)}$$

$$Cpss\ min = (Cpss\ max)(e^{-Kd\tau}) \qquad \text{(Eq. 38)}$$

$$Cpss\ min = \frac{\dfrac{(S)(F)(Dose)}{Vd}}{(1 - e^{-Kd\tau})} \times (e^{-Kd\tau}) \qquad \text{(Eq. 39)}$$

$$Cp^0 = \frac{(S)(F)(\text{Loading Dose})}{Vd} \qquad\qquad \text{(Eq. 40)}$$

$$\begin{aligned} Cp_1 &= (Cp^0)(e^{-Kdt_1}) \\ &= \frac{(S)(F)(\text{Loading Dose})}{Vd} \times (e^{-Kdt_1}) \end{aligned} \qquad \text{(Eq. 41)}$$

$$\begin{aligned} Cp_1 &= (Cpss\ ave)(e^{-Kdt_2}) \\ &= \frac{(S)(F)(\text{Dose}/\tau)}{Cl} \times (e^{-Kdt_2}) \end{aligned} \qquad \text{(Eq. 42)}$$

$$Cl_{Cr} = (100\ \text{ml/min})\left(\frac{1.0\ \text{mg/dl}}{SrCr_{ss}}\right) \qquad\qquad \text{(Eq. 43)}$$

$$Cl_{Cr} = (100\ \text{ml/min})\left(\frac{1.0\ \text{mg/dl}}{SrCr_{ss}}\right)\left(\frac{\text{Patient's BSA}}{1.73\text{m}^2}\right) \qquad \text{(Eq. 44)}$$

$$Cl_{Cr}\ \text{for males (ml/min/70 kg)} = \frac{98 - 0.8(\text{age} - 20)}{SrCr} \qquad \text{(Eq. 45)}$$

$$Cl_{Cr}\ \text{for females (ml/min/70 kg)} = 0.9\left[\frac{98 - 0.8(\text{age} - 20)}{SrCr}\right] \qquad \text{(Eq. 46)}$$

Amount of
Creatinine = (Urine Vol/24 hrs)(Urine Creatinine Conc) (Eq. 47)
Excreted

$$\text{Apparent Rate of Creatinine Production per Day (mg/kg/day)} = \frac{\text{Amount of Creatinine Excreted}}{\text{Patient's Weight}} \qquad \text{(Eq. 48)}$$

without congestive heart failure (70 kg):

Total
Digoxin (ml/min) = 57 ml/min + 1.02 (Cl_{Cr}) (Eq. 49)
Clearance

with congestive heart failure (70 kg):

Total
Digoxin (ml/min) = 23 ml/min + 0.88(Cl_{Cr}) (Eq. 50)
Clearance

$$\text{Digoxin Volume of Distribution (L/70 kg)} = 226 + \frac{298(Cl_{Cr})}{29 + Cl_{Cr}} \qquad \text{(Eq. 51)}$$

Digoxin
Volume of (L/70 kg) = 269 + 3.12(Cl_{Cr}) (Eq. 52)
Distribution

$$\text{Cpss max} = \frac{\frac{(S)(F)(Dose/t_{in})}{Cl} \times (1 - e^{-Kdt_{in}})}{(1 - e^{-Kd\tau})} \qquad \text{(Eq. 53)}$$

$$\text{Cpss min} = \text{Cpss max} \times e^{-Kd(\tau - t_{in})} \qquad \text{(Eq. 54)}$$

$$\text{Cpss min} = \frac{\frac{(S)(F)(Dose/t_{in})}{Cl} \times (1 - e^{Kdt_{in}})}{(1 - e^{-Kd\tau})} \times e^{-Kd(\tau - t_{in})} \qquad \text{(Eq. 55)}$$

$$v = \frac{(Vm)(s)}{Km + s} \qquad \text{(Eq. 56)}$$

$$(S)(F)(Dose/\tau) = \frac{(Vm)(Cpss)}{Km + Cpss} \qquad \text{(Eq. 57)}$$

$$Cpss = \frac{Km \times (S)(F)(Dose/\tau)}{Vm - (S)(F)(Dose/\tau)} \qquad \text{(Eq. 58)}$$

$$Cl = \frac{Vm}{Km + Cpss} \qquad \text{(Eq. 59)}$$

$$t\tfrac{1}{2} = \left(\frac{(0.693)(Vd)}{Vm}\right)(Km + Cpss) \qquad \text{(Eq. 60)}$$

$$Vm = \frac{(S)(F)(Dose/\tau)(Km + Cpss)}{Cpss} \qquad \text{(Eq. 61)}$$

$$Dose = \frac{(Vm)(Cpss)(\tau)}{(Km + Cpss)(S)(F)} \qquad \text{(Eq. 62)}$$

$$t = \frac{Km \times \ln\left(\frac{Cp^0}{Cp}\right) + (Cp^0 - Cp)}{\frac{Vm}{Vd}} \qquad \text{(Eq. 63)}$$

$$\text{Cp adjusted} = \frac{Cp'}{\left[(1 - \alpha)\left(0.44 \times \frac{P'}{P}\right)\right] + \alpha} \qquad \text{(Eq. 64)}$$

$$t_{90\%} = \frac{(Vm)(Vd)}{(Vm - R_A)^2}[2.303(Vm - 0.9R_A)] \qquad \text{(Eq. 65)}$$

APPENDIX III

GLOSSARY OF TERMS AND ABBREVIATIONS

Ab See Amount of Drug in the Body

Administration Rate (R_A) The average rate at which a drug is administered to the patient.

Alpha (α) (a) Fraction of the total plasma concentration which is free or unbound. (Eq. 5). (b) The initial half-life in a two compartment model, usually representing distribution. See Fig. 9.

Amount of Drug in the Body (Ab) The total amount of active drug which is in the body at any given time.

Average Steady State Concentration (Cpss ave) The average plasma drug concentration at steady state. (Eq. 31).

Beta (β) (a) Second decay half-life in a two compartment model, usually representing elimination. (b) The fraction of total plasma concentration which is bound to plasma proteins.

Bioavailability (F) The fraction of an administered dose which reaches the systemic circulation.

Body Surface Area (BSA) The surface area of a patient, as determined by weight and height. (Eq. 16). See Appendix I.

Bolus Dose A rapid intravenous injection of a dose.

BSA See Body Surface Area

Cl See Clearance

$Cl_{adjusted}$ Clearance of a patient which has been adjusted or altered for the presence of a disease state such as renal failure (Eq. 21) or heart failure.

Cl_{Cr} See Creatinine Clearance

Cl_m See Clearance, metabolic

Cl_r See Clearance, renal

Clearance (Cl_t or Cl) Total body clearance is a measure of how well a patient can metabolize or eliminate drug. It is used to calculate maintenance doses (Eq. 15) or average steady state plasma concentrations (Eq. 31).

Clearance, metabolic (Cl_m) A measure of how well the body can metabolize drugs. The major metabolic pathway is usually the liver.

Clearance, renal (Cl_r) A measure of how well the kidneys can excrete unchanged or unmetabolized drug. It is usually assumed to be proportional to creatinine clearance.

Cp See Plasma Concentration

Cp^0 The initial plasma concentration or the concentration at the beginning of a decay phase.

ΔCp Change in plasma concentration resulting from a bolus dose.

Cp free Unbound or free plasma concentration. (Eq. 8).

Cpss ave Average plasma concentration at steady state. (Eq. 31).

Cpss max Maximum or peak concentration at steady state, when a constant dose is administered at a constant dosing interval. (Eq. 36).

Cpss min The minimum or trough concentration at steady state when a constant dose is administered at a constant dosing interval. (Eq. 39).

Creatinine Clearance (Cl_{Cr}) A measure of the kidney's ability to eliminate creatinine from the body. Total renal function is usually assumed to be proportional to creatinine clearance.

Dosing Interval (τ) The time interval between doses when a drug is given intermittently.

e^{-Kdt} Fraction remaining at the end of a time interval.

$1 - e^{-Kdt}$ (a) Fraction lost during a dosing interval at steady state, if $t = \tau$. (b) Fraction of steady state achieved during a constant infusion "t" hours after starting the infusion.

Elimination Rate Constant (Kd) The fractional rate of drug loss from the body or the fraction of the volume of distribution which is cleared of drug during a time interval. (Eq. 23).

Elimination Rate (R_E) The amount of drug eliminated from the body during a time interval. (Eq. 12 and 13).

Extraction Ratio Fraction of drug which is removed from the blood or plasma as it passes through the eliminating organ.

F See Bioavailability

First-Pass Drug removed from the blood or plasma, following absorption from the gastrointestinal tract, before reaching the systemic circulation. See Fig. 2.

First-Order Elimination A process whereby the amount or concentration of drug in the body diminishes logarithmically over time. The rate of elimination is proportional to the drug concentration. See Fig. 15.

Half-life (t½) Time required for the plasma concentration to be reduced to one-half of the original value. (Eq. 27).

Half-life, alpha Initial decay half-life usually representing distribution of drug into the tissue or slowly equilibrating second compartment for a two compartmental model. See Fig. 9.

Half-life, beta Second decay half-life; usually represents the elimination half-life. Half-life, beta for most drugs can be calculated using the elimination rate constant. See Fig. 9. (Eq. 27).

Initial Volume of Distribution (Vi) Initial volume into which the drug rapidly equilibrates following an intravenous bolus injection.

Kd See Elimination Rate Constant

Kd$_{adjusted}$ Elimination rate constant which has been adjusted or altered for the presence of a disease state such as renal failure. (Eq. 25).

Km (Michaelis Menten Constant) Plasma concentration at which the rate of metabolism is occurring at half the maximum rate.

K_m The elimination rate constant resulting from the metabolic clearance and the volume of distribution (Cl_m/Vd).

K_r The elimination rate constant resulting from the renal clearance and the volume of distribution (Cl_r/Vd).

Linear Pharmacokinetics Assumes the elimination rate constant is not affected by plasma drug concentration and that the rate of drug elimination is directly proportional to the concentration of drug in plasma.

ln Natural logarithm using the base 2.718 rather than 10 which is used for the common logarithm or log.

Loading Dose   Initial total dose required to rapidly achieve a desired plasma concentration. (Eq. 10).

Maintenance Dose   The dose required to replace the amount of drug lost from the body so that a desired plasma concentration can be maintained. (Eq. 15).

One Compartment Model   Assumes that drug distributes equally to all areas of the body. Most drugs can be modeled this way if sampling during the initial distribution phase is avoided.

P or P'   Plasma protein concentration. P refers to the normal plasma protein concentration and P' refers to the plasma protein concentration of the specific patient.

Pharmacokinetics   Study of the absorption, distribution, metabolism and excretion of a drug and its metabolites in the body.

Plasma Concentration (Cp)   Concentration of drug in plasma. Usually refers to the total drug concentration and includes both the bound and free drug.

R_A   See Administration Rate

R_E   See Elimination Rate

S   See Salt Form

Salt Form (S)   Fraction of administered salt or ester form of the drug which is the active moiety.

SrCr   Serum Creatinine Concentration

Steady State   Steady state is achieved when the rate of drug administration is equal to the rate of drug elimination (Eq. 12 and 13). See Fig. 10.

$t_{1/2}$ See Half-life

Tau (τ)   See Dosing Interval

Tissue Concentration (Ct)   Concentration of drug in the tissue.

Tissue Volume of Distribution (Vt)   Apparent volume into which the drug appears to distribute following rapid equilibration with the initial volume of distribution.

Two Compartment Model   Comprised of an initial, rapidly equilibrating volume of distribution (Vi) and an apparent second, more slowly equilibrating volume of distribution (Vt).

Vd   See Volume of Distribution

Vi   See Initial Volume of Distribution

Vm   Maximum rate at which metabolism can occur.

Vt   See Tissue Volume of Distribution

Volume of Distribution (Vd)   The apparent volume required to account for all the drug in the body if it were present throughout the body in the same concentration as in the sample obtained from the plasma (Eq. 9).

References

1. Gibaldi M and Perrier D: *Pharmacokinetics,* Marcel Dekker, Inc., NY 1975
2. Winkle RA et al: Pharmacologic therapy of ventricular arrhythmias. Am J Card 36:629, 1975
3. Weinberger M et al: The relation of product formulation to absorption of oral theophylline. N Engl J Med 299:852, 1978
4. Powell JR et al: Theophylline disposition in acutely ill hospitalized patients. Am Rev Resp Dis 118:229, 1978
5. Koch-Weser J and Sellers EM: Binding of drugs to serum albumin. N Engl J Med 294:311, 1976
6. Sheiner, LB et al: Estimation of population characteristics of pharmacokinetic parameters from routine clinical data. J Pharmacokinetics Biopharm 5:445, 1977
7. Wilkinson G: A physiological approach to hepatic drug clearance. Clin Pharmacol Ther 18:377, 1975
8. Fremstad D et al: Increased plasma binding of quinidine after surgery. A preliminary report. Eur J Clin Pharmacol 10:441, 1976
9. Tucker GT et al: Binding of anilide-type local anesthetics in human plasma. Anesthesiology 33:287, 1970
10. Powers J and Sadee W: Determination of quinidine by high-performance liquid chromatography. Clin Chem 24:299, 1978
11. Drayer E: Pharmacologically active metabolites, therapeutic and toxic activities, plasma and urine data in man, accumulation in renal failure. Clin Pharmacokinetics 1:426, 1976
12. Jacobs MH et al: Clinical experience with theophylline: relationships between dosage, serum concentration and toxicity. JAMA 235:1983, 1976
13. Weinberger M et al: Intravenous aminophylline dosage: use of serum theophylline measurement for guidance. JAMA 235:2110, 1976
14. Lott RS and Hayton WL: Estimation of creatinine clearance from serum creatinine concentration: a review. Drug Intell Clin Pharm 12:140, 1978
15. Borga O et al: Plasma protein binding of basic drugs. Clin Pharmacol Ther 22:539, 1977
16. Barot MH et al: Individual variation in daily dosage requirements for phenytoin sodium in patients with epilepsy. Brit J Clin Pharm 6:267, 1978
17. Vogelstein B et al: The pharmacokinetics of amikacin in children. J Ped 91:333, 1977
18. Powell JR et al: The influence of cigarette smoking and sex on theophylline disposition. Am Rev Resp Dis 116:17, 1977
19. Pang SK and Rowland M: Hepatic clearance of drugs: I. Theoretical considerations of a "well-stirred" model and a "parallel tube" model. Influence of hepatic blood flow, plasma and blood cell binding and hepatocellular enzymatic activity on hepatic drug clearance. J Pharmacokinetics Biopharm 5:625, 1977
20. Adler DS et al: Hemodialysis of phenytoin in a uremic patient. Clin Pharmacol Ther 18:65, 1975

215

21. Aranda JV et al: Pharmacokinetic aspects of theophylline in premature newborns. N Engl J Med 295:413, 1976
22. Benowitz N: Clinical application of the pharmacokinetics of lidocaine, in *Cardiovascular Drug Therapy,* K Melmon, Ed. FM Davis, Philadelphia 1974, pp 77–101
23. Boyer RW et al: Pharmacokinetics of lidocaine in man. Clin Pharmacol Ther 12:105, 1971
24. Chiou WL et al: Pharmacokinetics of creatinine in man and its implications in the monitoring of renal function and in dosage regimen modifications in patients with renal insufficiency. J Clin Pharmacol 15:427, 1975
25. Chow MS et al: Pharmacokinetic data and drug monitoring: Antibiotics and antiarrhythmics. J Clin Pharmacol 15:405, 1975
26. Cramer G and Isakson B: Quantitative determination of quinidine in plasma. Scand J Clin Lab Invest 15:553, 1963
27. Dettli L: Individualization of drug dosage in patients with renal disease. Med Clin N Am 58:977, 1974
28. Gibaldi M and Perrier D: Drug distribution and renal failure. J Clin Pharmacol 12:201, 1972
29. Gibson TP: Acetylation of procainamide in man and its relationship to isonicotinic acid-hydrazide acetylation phenotype. Clin Pharmacol Ther 17:395, 1975
30. Goldman R: Creatinine excretion in renal failure. Proc Soc Exp Biol Med 85:446, 1954
31. Huffman DH et al: Absorption of digoxin from different oral preparations in normal subjects during steady state. Clin Pharmacol Ther 16:310, 1974
32. Jelliffe RW: Creatinine clearance: Bedside estimate. Ann Intern Med 70:604, 1973
33. Jusko WJ et al: Pharmacokinetic design of digoxin dosage regimens in relation to renal function. J Clin Pharmacol 14:525, 1974
34. Kassirer JP: Clinical evaluation of kidney function-glomerular function. N Engl J Med 285:385, 1971
35. Kessler KM et al: Quinidine elimination in patients with congestive heart failure or poor renal function. N Engl J Med 290:706, 1974
36. Koch-Weser J et al: Influence of serum digoxin concentration measurements on frequency of digitoxicity. Clin Pharmacol Ther 16:284, 1974
37. Mitenko PA and Ogilvie RI: Rapidly achieved plasma concentration plateaus, with observation on theophylline kinetics. Clin Pharmacol Ther 13:329, 1972
38. Mitenko PA and Ogilvie RI: Rational intravenous doses of theophylline. N Engl J Med 289:600, 1973
39. Niles AS and Shand DG: Clinical pharmacology of propranolol. Circ 52:6, 1975
40. Odar-Cedarlof I, Borga O et al: Kinetics of diphenylhydantoin in uremic patients: consequence of decreased protein binding. Eur J Clin Pharmacol 7:31, 1974
41. Pagliaro LA et al: Critical compilation of terminal half-lives, percent excreted unchanged, and changes of half-life in renal and hepatic dysfunction for studies in humans with references. J Pharmacokinetics Biopharm 3:333, 1975
42. Reuning RH et al: Role of pharmacokinetics in drug dosage adjustment: I. Pharmacologic effect kinetics and apparent volume of distribution of digoxin. J Clin Pharmacol 13:127, 1973
43. Rowland M: Drug administration and regimens, in *Clinical Pharmacology and Therapeutics,* 2nd Edit. K Melmon and H Morelli, Eds. MacMillan, New York, 1978, pp 25–70
44. Documentia Geigy: *Scientific Tables,* 7th Edit., Diem K and Lentner C, Eds. Ciba-Geigy, Ltd., Switzerland, 1972

45. Sheiner LB et al: Instructional goals for physicians in the use of blood level data and the contribution of computers. Clin Pharmacol Ther 16:260, 1974

46. Shirkey HC: *Posology in Pediatric Therapy,* 5th Edit. Shirkey HC, Ed. Mosby, St. Louis, 1972. p 32

47. Siersback-Nielson K et al: Rapid evaluation of creatinine clearance (letter). Lancet 1:1133, 1971

48. Thompson PD: Lidocaine pharmacokinetics in advanced heart failure, liver disease, and renal failure in humans. Ann Intern Med 78:499, 1973

49. Wagner JG: *Biopharmaceutics and Relevant Pharmacokinetics.* Drug Intelligence Publications, Illinois, 1971. pp 18–25

50. FDA Drug Bulletin Vol. 10, Feb. 1980.

51. Walsh FM et al: Significance of non-steady state serum digoxin concentrations. Am J Clin Pathol 63:446, 1975

52. Welling PG et al: Prediction of drug dosage in patients with renal failure using data derived from normal subjects. Clin Pharmacol Ther 18:45, 1975

53. Shapiro W et al: Relationship of plasma digitoxin and digoxin to cardiac response following intravenous digitalization in man. Circ 42:1065, 1970

54. Smith TW: Digitalis toxicity: epidemiology and clinical use of serum concentration measurements. Am J Med 58:470, 1975

55. Smith TW and Haber E: Digoxin intoxication: the relationship of clinical presentation to serum digoxin concentration. J Clin Invest 49:2377, 1970

56. Ogilvie RI and Ruedy J: An educational program in digitalis therapy. JAMA 222:50, 1972

57. Lisalo E: Clinical pharmacokinetics of digoxin. Clin Pharmacokinetics 2:1, 1977

58. Koup JR et al: Digoxin pharmacokinetics: Role of renal failure in dosage regimen design. Clin Pharmacol Ther 18:9, 1975

59. Jusko WJ and Weintraub M: Myocardial distribution of digoxin and renal function. Clin Pharmacol Ther 16:449, 1974

60. Wagner JG: Loading and maintenance doses of digoxin in patients with normal renal function and those with severely impaired renal function. J Clin Pharmacol 14:329, 1974

61. Ohnhaus EE et al: Protein binding of digoxin in human serum. Eur J Clin Pharmacol 5:34, 1972

62. Jusko WJ: Clinical pharmacokinetics of digoxin. *Clinical Pharmacokinetics: A Symposium.* G. Levy, Ed. Am Pharm Assoc, Acad Pharm Sci, p 31 1974

63. Koup JR et al: Pharmacokinetics of digoxin in normal subjects after intravenous bolus and infusion doses. J Pharmacokinetics Biopharm 3:181, 1975

64. Weintraub M et al: Compliance as a determinant of serum digoxin concentration. JAMA 224:481, 1973

65. Sheiner LB et al: Modeling of individual pharmacokinetics for computer-aided drug dosage. Comp Biomed Res 5:441, 1972

66. Kramer WG et al: Pharmacokinetics of digoxin: comparison of a two and a three compartment model in man. J Pharmacokinetics Biopharm 2:299, 1974

67. Lader S et al: The measurement of plasma digoxin concentrations: a comparison of two methods. Eur J Clin Pharmacol 5:22, 1972

68. Smith TW et al: Clinical value of the radioimmunoassay of the digitalis glycosides. Pharmacological Rev 25:219, 1973

69. Silber B et al: Associated digoxin radioimmunoassay interference. Clin Chem 25:48, 1979

70. Doherty et al: Digoxin metabolism in hypo- and hyperthyroidism. Ann Intern Med 64:489, 1966
71. Lawrence JR: Digoxin kinetics in patients with thyroid dysfunction. Clin Pharmacol Ther 22:7, 1977
72. Croxson MS and Ibbertson HK: Serum digoxin in patients with thyroid disease. Brit Med J 3:566, 1975
73. Luchi RJ and Gruber JW: Unusually large digitalis requirements. Am J Med 45:322, 1968
74. Ackerman GL et al: Peritoneal and hemodialysis of tritiated digoxin. Ann Int Med 67:4:718, 1967
75. Ejvinsson G: Effect of quinidine on plasma concentrations of digoxin. Brit Med J 279, 1978
76. Leahey EB, Jr et al: Interactions between quinidine and digoxin. JAMA 240:533, 1978
77. Koch-Weser J: Pharmacokinetics of procainamide in man. Ann NY Acad Sci 169:370, 1971
78. Koch-Weser J and Klein SW: Procainamide dosage schedules, plasma concentrations and clinical effects. JAMA 215:1454, 1971
79. Noone P et al: Experience in monitoring gentamicin therapy during treatment of serious gram-negative sepsis. Brit Med J 1:477, 1974
80. Jackson GG and Riff LF: Pseudomonas bacteremia: Pharmacologic and other basis for failure of treatment with gentamicin. J Infect Dis 124(Suppl):185, 1971
81. Klastersky J et al: Antibacterial activity in serum and urine as a therapeutic guide in bacterial infections. J Infect Dis 129:187, 1974
82. Dahlgren JG et al: Gentamicin blood levels: a guide to nephrotoxicity. Antimicrob Agents Chemother 8:58, 1975
83. Cox CE: Gentamicin: a new aminoglycoside antibiotic: Clinical and laboratory studies in urinary tract infections. J Infect Dis 119:486, 1969
84. Jackson GG and Arcieri G: Ototoxicity of gentamicin in man: A survey and controlled analysis of clinical experience in the United States. J Infect Dis 124(Suppl):130, 1971
85. Goodman EL et al: Prospective comparative study of variable dosage and variable frequency regimens for administrations of gentamicin, Antimicrob Agents Chemother 8:434, 1975
86. Mawer GE: Prescribing aids for gentamicin. Brit J Clin Pharmacol 1:45, 1974
87. Black RS et al: Ototoxicity of amikacin. Antimicrob Agents Chemother 9:956, 1976
88. Reiner NE et al: Nephrotoxicity of gentamicin and tobramycin in dogs on a continuous or once daily intravenous injection. Antimicrob Agents Chemother 4(Suppl A):85, 1978
89. Federspil P et al: Pharmacokinetics and ototoxicity of gentamicin, tobramycin, and amikacin. J Infect Dis 134:(suppl):200 1976
90. Wilfret JN et al: Renal insufficiency associated with gentamicin therapy. J Infect Dis 124(Suppl):148, 1971
91. Gyselynek AM et al: Pharmacokinetics of gentamicin: distribution and plasma and renal clearance. J Infect Dis 124(Suppl):70, 1971
92. Christopher TG et al: Gentamicin pharmacokinetics during hemodialysis. Kidney Intl 6:38, 1974
93. Danish M et al: Pharmacokinetics of gentamicin and kanamicin during hemodialysis. Antimicrob Agents Chemother 6:841, 1974

94. Barza M et al: Predictability of blood levels of gentamicin in man. J Infect Dis 132:165, 1975
95. Sawchuck RJ and Zaske DE: Pharmacokinetics of dosing regimens which utilize multiple intravenous infusions: gentamicin in burn patients. J Pharmacokinetics Biopharm 4:183, 1976
96. Regamey C et al: Comparative pharmacokinetics of tobramicin and gentamicin. Clin Pharmacol Ther 14:396, 1973
97. Hull JH and Sarubbi FA: Gentamicin serum concentrations: pharmacokinetic predictions. Ann Int Med 85:183, 1976
98. Schentag JJ and Jusko WJ: Renal clearance and tissue accumulation of gentamicin. Clin Pharmacol Ther 22:364, 1977
99. Mendelson J et al: Safety of bolus administration of gentamicin. Antimicrob Agents Chemother 9:633, 1976
100. Lynn KL et al: Gentamicin by intravenous bolus injections. New Zealand Med J 80:442, 1977
101. Schentag JJ et al: Tissue persistence of gentamicin in man. JAMA 238:327, 1977
102. Colburn WA et al: A model for the prospective identification of the prenephrotoxic state during gentamicin therapy. J Pharmacokinetics Biopharm 6:179, 1978
103. Holt HA et al: Interactions between aminoglycoside antibiotics and carbenicillin or ticarcillin. Infect 4:107, 1976
104. Ervin FR et al: Inactivation of gentamicin by penicillins in patients with renal failure. Antimicrob Agents Chemother 9:1004, 1976
105. Weibert RT and Keane WF: Carbinicillin-gentamicin interaction in acute renal failure. Am J Hosp Pharm 34:1137, 1977
106. Riff L and Jackson GG: Laboratory and clinical conditions for gentamicin inactivation by carbenicillin. Arch Int Med 130:887, 1972
107. Siber GR et al: Pharmacokinetics of gentamicin in children and adults. J Infect Dis 132:637, 1975
108. Schultze RG: Possible nephrotoxicity of gentamicin. J Infect Dis 124(Suppl): 145, 1971
109. Kleinknecht D et al: Acute renal failure after high doses of gentamicin and cephalothin. Lancet 7812:1129, 1973
110. Reguer L et al: Pharmacokinetics of amikacin during hemodialysis and peritoneal dialysis. Antimicrob Agents Chemother 11:214, 1977
111. Christopher TG et al: Hemodializer clearance of gentamicin, kanamycin, tobramycin, amikacin, ethambutol, procainamide, and flucytosine with a technique for planning therapy. J Pharmacokinetics Biopharm 4:427, 1976
112. Gailiunas, P et al: Vestibular toxicity of gentamicin: incidence in patients receiving long-term hemodialysis therapy. Arch Int Med 138:1621, 1978
113. Gary NE: Peritoneal clearance and removal of gentamicin. J Infect Dis 124(Suppl):96, 1971
114. Halprin BA et al: Clearance of gentamicin during hemodialysis: A comparison of four artificial kidneys. J Infect Dis 133:627, 1976
115. Kaiser AB: Aminoglycoside therapy of gram-negative bacillary meningitis. N Engl J Med 293:1215, 1975
116. Rahal JJ et al: Combined intrathecal and intramuscular gentamicin for gram-negative meningitis. New Engl J Med 290:1394, 1974
117. Sokolow M and Ball RE: Factors influencing conversion of chronic atrial fibrillation with special reference to serum quinidine concentration. Circ 14:568, 1956

118. Hartel G and Harjanne A: Comparisons of two methods for quinidine determination and chromatographic analysis of the difference. Clin Chim Acta 23:124, 1969
119. Conn HL and Luchi RJ: Some cellular and metabolic considerations relating to the action of quinidine as a prototype antiarrhythmic agent. Am J Med 37:685, 1969
120. Di Bonna GF: Measurement of plasma quinidine (letter). N Engl J Med 290:1325, 1974
121. Conrad KA et al: Pharmacokinetic studies of quinidine in patients with arrhythmias. Circ 55:1, 1977
122. Ueda CT and Dzindzio BS: Quinidine kinetics in congestive failure. Clin Pharmacol Ther 23:158, 1978
123. Thompson GW: Quinidine as a cause of sudden death. Circ 14:757, 1956
124. Wetherbee DG et al: Ventricular tachycardia following the administration of quinidine. Am Heart J 43:89, 1952
125. Greenblatt DJ et al: Pharmacokinetics of parenteral quinidine in humans. (Abs.) Clin Pharmacol Ther 21:105, 1977
126. Kessler KM: Blood collection techniques, heparin, and quinidine protein binding. Clin Pharmacol Ther 25:204, 1979
127. Kessler KM et al: Quinidine pharmacokinetics in patients with cirrhosis, or receiving propranolol. Am Heart J 96:627, 1978
128. Staprans I and Felts JM: The effect of alpha I acid glycoprotein on triglyceride metabolism in nephrotic syndrome. Biochem Biophys Res Commun 79:1272, 1977
129. Bolme P and Otto U: Dose-dependence of the pharmacokinetics of quinidine. Eur J Clin Pharmacol 12:73, 1977
130. Gianelly R et al: Effect of lidocaine on ventricular arrhythmias in patients with coronary heart disease. N Engl J Med 277:1215, 1967
131. Jewett DE et al: Lidocaine in the management of arrhythmias after acute myocardial infarction. Lancet 1:266, 1968
132. Seldon R and Sasahara AA: Central nervous system toxicity induced by lidocaine. JAMA 202:908, 1967
133. Stannard M et al: Hemodynamic effects of lidocaine in acute myocardial infarction. Brit Med J 2:468, 1968
134. Le Lorier J et al: Pharmacokinetics of lidocaine after prolonged intravenous infusions in uncomplicated myocardial infarction. Ann Int Med 87:700, 1977
135. Collingsworth KA et al: Pharmacokinetics and metabolism of lidocaine in patients with renal failure. Clin Pharmacol Ther 18:59, 1975
136. Strong JM et al: Pharmacological activity, metabolism, and pharmacokinetics of glycinexylidide. Clin Pharmacol Ther 17:184, 1975
137. Anderson JL et al: Anti-arrhythmic drugs: clinical pharmacology and therapeutic uses. Drugs 15:271, 1978
138. Cheng TO and Wadhwa K: Sinus standstill following intravenous lidocaine administration. JAMA 223:790, 1973
139. Zito RA and Reid P: Lidocaine kinetics predicted by indocyanine green clearance. N Engl J Med 298:1160, 1978
140. Prescott LF et al: Impaired lignocaine metabolism in patients with myocardial infarction and cardiac failure. Brit Med J 1:939, 1976
141. Prescott LF and Nimmo J: Plasma lidocaine concentrations during and after prolonged infusion in patients with myocardial infarction. *Lidocaine in the Treatment of Ventricular Arrhythmias.* Scott DB and Julian DG, Eds. Edinburgh and Livingstone, Ltd. 1971, 168

142. Buchthal F et al: Relation of EEG and seizures to phenobarbital in serum. Arch Neurol 19:567, 1968
143. Plaa GL and Hine CH: Hydantoin and barbiturate blood levels observed in epileptics. Arch Int Pharmacodyn Ther 128:375, 1960
144. Sunshine I: Chemical evidence of tolerance to phenobarbital. J Lab Clin Med 50:127, 1957
145. Baselt RC et al: Therapeutic and toxic concentrations of more than 100 toxicologically significant drugs in blood, plasma, or serum: a tabulation. Clin Chem 21:44, 1975
146. Kennedy AC et al: Successful treatment of three cases of very severe barbiturate poisoning. Lancet 1:995, 1969
147. Havidberg E and Dam M: Clinical pharmacokinetics of anticonvulsants. Clin Pharmacokinetics 1:161, 1976
148. Alvin J et al: The effect of liver disease in man on the disposition of phenobarbital. J Pharmacol Exper Ther 192:224, 1975
149. Svensmark O and Bachthal F: Accumulation of phenobarbital in man. Epilepsia 4:199, 1963
150. Van Der Kleijn E et al: Clinical pharmacokinetics in monitoring chronic medications with antiepileptic drugs in Clinical Pharmacology of Anti-epileptic Drugs. Schneider, Janz, Gardner-Thorpe, Meinard, and Sherwin, Eds. Springer-Verlag, Berlin 1975 pp 11–33
151. Linton AL et al: Methods of forced diuresis and its application in barbiturate poisoning. Lancet 2:377, 1967
152. Henderson LW and Merrill JP: Treatment of barbiturate intoxication. Ann Int Med 64:876, 1966
153. Waddell WJ and Butler TC: The distribution of phenobarbital. J Clin Invest 36:1217, 1957
154. Houghton GW et al: Brain concentrations of phenytoin, phenobarbitone, and primidone in epileptic patients. Eur J Clin Pharmacol 9:73, 1975
155. Ueda CT et al: Absolute quinidine bioavailability. Clin Pharmacol Ther 20:260, 1976
156. Ueda CT et al: Disposition of quinidine. Clin Pharmacol Ther 19:30, 1976
157. Jelliffe RW et al: Reduction of digitalis toxicity by computer assisted glycoside dosage regimens. Ann Int Med 77:891, 1972
158. Echeverria P et al: Age dependent dose-response to gentamicin. J Ped 87:805, 1975
159. Bierman CW et al: Acute and chronic therapy in exercise induced bronchospasm. Ped 60:845, 1977
160. Jenne JW: Pharmacokinetics of theophylline: application to adjustment of the clinical dose of aminophylline. Clin Pharmacol Ther 13:349, 1972
161. Piafsky KM and Ogilvie RI: Dosage of theophylline in bronchial asthma. N Engl J Med 292:1218, 1975
162. Zillich CW et al: Theophylline-induced seizures in adults. Ann Int Med 82:784, 1975
163. Yarnell PR and Chu NS: Focal seizures and aminophylline. Neurology 25:819, 1975
164. Mitenko PA and Ogilvie RI: Pharmacokinetics of intravenous theophylline. Clin Pharmacol Ther 14:509, 1972
165. Gal P et al: Theophylline disposition in obesity. Clin Pharmacol Ther 23:438, 1978
166. Hunt SN et al: Effects of smoking on theophylline disposition. Clin Pharmacol Ther 19:546, 1976

167. Jenne JW et al: Apparent theophylline half-life fluctuations during treatment of acute left ventricular failure. Am J Hosp Pharm 34:408, 1977

168. Jusko WJ et al: Intravenous theophylline therapy: nomogram guideline. Ann Int Med 86:400, 1977

169. Piafsky KM et al: Theophylline kinetics in acute pulmonary edema. Clin Pharmacol Ther 21:310, 1977

170. Piafsky KM et al: Theophylline disposition in patients with hepatic cirrhosis. N Engl J Med 296:1495, 1977

171. Weinberger M et al: Inhibition of theophylline clearance by triacetyloleandomycin. J Allergy Clin Immunol 59:228, 1977

172. Kozak RP et al: Administration of erythromycin to patients on theophylline. J Allergy Clin Immunol 16:149, 1977

173. Landay RA: Effect of phenobarbital on theophylline disposition. J Allergy Immunol 62:27, 1978

174. Piafsky KM et al: Effect of phenobarbital on the disposition of intravenous theophylline. Clin Pharmacol Ther 22:336, 1977

175. Levy G et al: Pharmacokinetic analysis of the effect of theophylline on pulmonary function in asthmatic children. J Pediatr 86:789, 1978

176. Maselli R et al: Pharmacologic effect of intravenously administered aminophylline in asthmatic children. J Pediatr 76:777, 1970

177. Wyatt R et al: Oral theophylline dosage for the management of chronic asthma. J Pediatr 92:125, 1978

178. Lee WK et al: Antiarrhythmic efficacy of N-acetylprocainamide in patients with premature ventricular contractions. Clin Pharmacol Ther 19:508, 1976

179. Elson J et al: Antiarrhythmic potency of N-acetylprocainamide. Clin Pharmacol Ther 17:134, 1975

180. Atkinson AJ Jr. et al: Dose ranging trial of N-acetylprocainamide in patients with premature ventricular contractions. Clin Pharmacol Ther 21:575, 1977

181. Gibson TP et al: Kinetics of procainamide and N-acetylprocainamide in renal failure. Kidney Intl 12:422, 1977

182. Manion CV et al: Absorption kinetics of procainamide in humans. J Pharm Sci 66:981, 1977

183. Galeazzi RL et al: Relationship between the pharmacokinetics and pharmacodymanics of procainamide. Clin Pharmacol Ther 20:278, 1976

184. Giardina EV and Heissenbuttel RH: Intermittent intravenous procainamide to treat ventricular arrhythmias. Ann Int Med 78:183, 1973

185. Lima JJ et al: Pharmacokinetic approach to intravenous procainamide therapy. Eur J Clin Pharmacol 13:303, 1978

186. Giardina EV et al: Metabolism of procainamide in normal and cardiac subjects. Clin Pharmacol Ther 19:339, 1976

187. Bagwell EE et al: Correlation of the electrophysiological and antiarrhythmic properties of the N-acetyl metabolite of procainamide with plasma and tissue drug concentration in the dog. J Pharmacol Exper Ther 197:38, 1976

188. Karlsson E et al: Acetylation of procainamide in man studied with a new gas chromatographic method. Brit J Pharmacol 1:467, 1974

189. Reidenberg MM et al: Polymorphic acetylation of procainamide in man. Clin Pharmacol Ther 17:722, 1975

190. Drayer DE et al: N-acetylprocainamide: an active metabolite of procainamide. Proc Soc Exper Biol Med 146:358, 1974

191. Vesell JM et al: Recent progress in pharmacogenetics. Advances Pharm Chemother 7:1, 1969

192. Dreyfuss J: Metabolism of procainamide in rhesus monkey and man. Clin Pharmacol Ther 13:366, 1972
193. Strong JM et al: Pharmacokinetics in man of the N-acetylated metabolite of procainamide. J Pharmacokinetics Biopharm 3:223, 1975
194. Strong JM et al: Absolute bioavailability in man of N-acetylprocainamide determined by a novel stable isotope method. Clin Pharmacol Ther 18:613, 1975
195. Gibson TP et al: N-acetylprocainamide levels in patients with end-stage renal failure. Clin Pharmacol Ther 19:206, 1976
196. Glazko AJ et al: Metabolic disposition of diphenylhydantoin in normal human subjects following intravenous administration. Clin Pharmacol Ther 10:498, 1969
197. Gugler R et al: Phenytoin: pharmacokinetics and bioavailability. Clin Pharmacol Ther 19:135, 1976
198. Albert KS: Bioavailability of diphenylhydantoin. Clin Pharmacol Ther 16:272, 1974
199. Bigger JT et al: Relationship between the plasma level of diphenylhydantoin sodium and its cardiac antiarrhythmic effects. Circ 38:363, 1968
200. Louis S et al: The cardiocirculatory changes caused by intravenous dilantin and its solvent. Amer Heart J 74:523, 1967
201. Wilder BJ et al: Plasma diphenylhydantoin levels after loading and maintenance doses. Clin Pharmacol Ther 14:797, 1973
202. Kutt H et al: Diphenylhydantoin metabolism, blood levels and toxicity. Arch Neurol 11:642, 1964
203. Bochner F et al: Effects of dosage increments on blood phenytoin concentrations. J Neurol Neurosurg Psych 35:873, 1972
204. Arnold K et al: The rate of decline of diphenylhydantoin in human plasma. Clin Pharmacol Ther 11:121, 1970
205. Houghton GW and Richens A: Rate of elimination of tracer doses of phenytoin at different steady state serum phenytoin concentrations in epileptic patients. Brit J Clin Pharmacol 1:155, 1974
206. Lund L et al: Pharmacokinetics of single and multiple doses of phenytoin in man. Eur J Clin Pharmacol 7:81, 1974
207. Mawer GE et al: Phenytoin dose adjustments in epileptic patients. Brit J Clin Pharmacol 1:163, 1974
208. Lambie DG et al: Therapeutic and pharmacokinetic effects of increasing phenytoin in chronic epileptics on multiple drug therapy. Lancet 2:386, 1976
209. Richens A: A study of the pharmacokinetics of phenytoin (diphenylhydantoin) in epileptic patients, and the development of a nomogram for making dose increments. Epilepsia 16:627, 1975
210. Ludden TM et al: Individualization of phenytoin dosage regimens. Clin Pharmacol Ther 21:287, 1977
211. Martin E et al: The clinical pharmacokinetics of phenytoin. J Pharmacokinetics Biopharm 5:579, 1977
212. Mullen PW: Optimal phenytoin therapy: a new technique for individualizing dosage. Clin Pharmacol Ther 23:228, 1978
213. Atkinson AJ and Shaw JM: Pharmacokinetic study of a patient with diphenylhydantoin toxicity. Clin Pharmacol Ther 14:521, 1973
214. Lund L et al: Plasma protein binding of diphenylhydantoin in patients with epilepsy. Clin Pharmacol Ther 13:196, 1972
215. Reidenberg MM et al: Protein binding of diphenylhydantoin and desmethylimipramine in plasma from patients with poor renal function. N Engl J Med 285:264, 1971

216. Odar-Cedarlof I: Plasma protein binding of phenytoin and warfarin in patients undergoing renal transplantation. Clin Pharmacokinetics 2:147, 1977
217. Reidenberg MM: The binding of drugs to plasma proteins and the interpretation of measurements of plasma concentrations of drugs in patients with poor renal function. Am J Med 62:466, 1977
218. Morselli PL et al: Interaction between phenobarbital and DPH in animals and epileptic patients. Ann NY Acad Sci 169, 1971
219. Kutt H et al: Depression of parahydroxylation of diphenylhydantoin by antituberculosis chemotherapy. Neurology 16:594, 1966
220. Rose JQ et al: Intoxication caused by interaction of chloramphenicol and phenytoin. JAMA 237:2630, 1977
221. Kutt H et al: Inhibition of diphenylhydantoin metabolism in rats and in rat liver microsomes by antitubercular drugs. Neurology 18:706, 1968
222. Wilensky AJ et al: Inadequate serum levels after intramuscular administration of diphenylhydantoin. Neurology 23:318, 1973
223. Wilder BJ et al: A method for shifting from oral to intramuscular diphenylhydantoin administration. Clin Pharmacol Ther 16:507, 1974
224. Blouin RA et al: Tobramycin pharmacokinetics in morbidly obese patients. Clin Pharmacol Ther 26:508, 1979
225. Bauer LA et al: Amikacin pharmacokinetics in morbidly obese patients. Am J Hosp Pharm 37:519, 1980
226. Hager DW et al: Digoxin-quinidine interaction. N Engl J Med 300:1238, 1979
227. Powell JR et al: Quinidine-digoxin interaction. N Engl J Med 302:176, 1980
228. Doering W: Quinidine-digoxin interaction. N Engl J Med 301:400, 1979
229. Pfeifer HJ et al: Effects of three antibiotics on theophylline kinetics. Clin Pharmacol Ther 26:36, 1979
230. Jusko WJ et al: Nonlinear assessment of phenytoin bioavailability. J Pharmacokin Biopharm 4:327, 1976
231. Richens A and Dunlop A: Serum phenytoin levels in the management of epilepsy. Lancet 2:247, 1975

Index